Twenty-Four More in Acupuncture

SECOND IN A SERIES

ADVANCED PRINCIPLES AND TECHNIQUES

譚 特 夫

RICHARD TAN, O.M.D., L.Ac.

and

STEPHEN C. RUSH, L.Ac.

SAN DIEGO, CALIFORNIA

For information contact Richard Tan, O.M.D., L.Ac.
4550 Kearny Villa Rd., Ste. 107, San Diego, CA 92123.

Editors: Stephen Rush, Cheryl Warnke, Mary Kanable
Composition and Illustrations: Cheryl Warnke

Printed in San Diego, California

Acknowledgments

————•◆•————

We would like to thank the following people
for their contributions to the development of
Twenty-Four More in Acupuncture.

Cheryl Warnke, for her excellent artwork, editing,
typesetting, design, and emotional support.

Mary Kanable, for her copy editing and proofreading.

Dr. Tan's wife Fang Fang, and his family, for their
understanding and patience throughout the many late
night and weekend meetings this book required.

All of our patients, from whom we have each
learned a great deal.

Contents

Chapter 1

To Our Readers

———•◆•———

After three years in print, *Twelve and Twelve in Acupuncture* has been favorably received by virtually all of our readers. We have received many letters, faxes, phone calls, and other communications regarding our first book's utility in the clinic. Apparently, our book has found a somewhat overlooked niche in the body of acupuncture literature that we had long suspected was there, waiting to be filled. Another possibility is that we have succeeded in creating a niche for our work. That may very well be true. However, rather than ruminating in print over these theoretical matters, we prefer remaining consistent with our nuts-and-bolts style as established in *Twelve and Twelve*. We really aren't interested in contemplation of such a "chicken or egg" paradigm at the present. Our main concern is to provide our colleagues with useful and effective clinical techniques in acupuncture. We don't think of our workbook style of presentation as stripped-down, but as accessible, easy to use. And we are more confident than ever of the potential our information has to significantly improve the clinical efficacy of any practice. Judging from the feedback we have received, the vast majority of you agree with this approach.

Over the past three years, we have developed many new applications and techniques. After careful testing, we are prepared to offer this new information to our readers to try for themselves.

1

In *Twelve and Twelve*, we were the first to publish information in English about twelve of Master Tong's more effective points, as well as twelve unique applications of "regular" meridian points. Most of the information encountered by the reader in *Twenty-Four More* will also constitute the first time it has been seen in print. The only exceptions we know of are in the case of two of our articles that were accepted for publication in the now-defunct *Yuin Journal*, and only one of these actually made it into print before the journal folded. A few of the point applications and techniques described in *Twenty-Four More* are more or less generally known in the profession, but in our opinion are either incorrectly applied, or underutilized. We have included them here because we feel that they are so effective in distal application that it would be remiss of us to leave them out. In many instances the way we use these points differs from the norm, consequently, it is felt that the reader is likely to benefit from this seeming redundancy. In this book, the reader will not find any extra points from Master Tong or any other source. But, for the most part will encounter familiar regular channel points, along with our largely unique discoveries concerning their application.

As we assembled the material for inclusion in this latest offering, we adhered to the same criteria that we used for *Twelve and Twelve*. As in our first book, the points and techniques in *Twenty-Four More* conform to three requirements:

1) That results be obtained in a noticeable fashion within seconds of application, or within a minute or two at the longest.

2) That all techniques be comprised of "distal" treatment techniques that do not, in most cases, require any local needling to supplement their effect.

3) That the number of needles required in order to perform an effective treatment be minimal—usually fewer than six.

The numerous case studies we have included illustrate the desirability of these features in what we hope, is a thorough manner.

Since the publication of *Twelve and Twelve*, we have been invited to attend conferences and seminars throughout the United States as well as Europe. Dr. Tan's method of presenting our material in a lecture situation, leaning heavily on actual patient demonstrations, is much appreciated by audiences wherever we go. It is also under such circumstances that Dr. Tan is able to more fully elaborate on the theoretical connections between our method and his personal interpretation of I-Ching theory. However, we try to be careful not to fall into the trap of excessive complexity that so many acupuncture theoreticians succumbed to in Traditional Chinese Medicine's past. On more than one occasion confusion was the main effect when one elaborate theory would only be found to contradict yet another equally intricate system. Therefore, we believe that the best theory is one that is the simplest and the easiest to apply, while also yielding the most consistently high degree of positive results. Even so, we hope to satisfy our readers theoretical appetite in the future with a publication dedicated solely to that. Although it will amount to a sort of inverse of our previous work, we are sure you will find it of interest.

Many of our readers call or fax us with questions concerning difficult cases. At times, the demand for our replies exceeds the time we have available. To address this need, we are presently developing plans for a membership-based organization and journal. All members will be welcome to present cases of their own, with an open discussion by the entire group to follow. Some of this will be conducted in print, but we would also like to facilitate open forum-style meetings in which members could participate directly. Perhaps a computer bulletin board could also be established. (Dr. Tan is also a systems analyst with many years of experience in the computer field.)

In short, we really would like to discuss clinically relevant issues with our colleagues in an atmosphere of openness and professionalism. Additionally, we also want to avoid as much as possible involvement with any of the many political factions and institutions which seem to be battling over the future of our profession. While others may be drawn to the political struggle, we feel that the best way that we as individuals can contribute to the field is by helping to make acupuncturists better practitioners in their clinics. No matter which way you look at it, the more effective acupuncturists are as a group, the more valued the profession will be.

Chapter 2

Using
Twenty–Four More

———•◆•———

We have provided two sets of indices for *Twenty-Four More* that will, as was also hopefully the case with *Twelve and Twelve*, make the information more easily accessible. *Index 1* lists the points according to nomenclature, as well as all references to them throughout the book. *Index 2* alphabetically lists symptoms covered in the point indications and case studies.

Point Locations: All of the points found in *Twenty-Four More* are referred to by the nomenclature assigned them in the Beijing textbook *Chinese Acupuncture and Moxibustion*. Even though it is a universally recognized text in the profession, we have included point location descriptions as well as illustrations for the benefit of any of our readers who are non-acupuncturists. In addition, for those readers who are acupuncturists and are in fact using needles, it is assumed that they all are familiar with the established needling depths and all other precautions that must be observed with needle treatment. Practitioners reading this book who are not legally qualified to perform acupuncture, must not try any of the needling techniques described herein. In every state that we know of, such an unlicensed attempt at acupuncture constitutes a crime. Also, the point location and functions pages are designed for quick reference use: the related case studies contain much vital information concerning their correct application. Before attempting to treat a patient with these points, please read the case studies carefully.

Another term that all acupuncturists are familiar with is the Chinese phrase *ah shi*. The term ah shi simply denotes a sensitive spot that is suitable for treatment, even though its location may not be exactly that of an established well-known acupuncture point. As such, the use of ah shi points is important in the treatment protocol of many acupuncture styles.

Qi Sensation: With our method, needling for the Qi Sensation definitely produces a higher rate of efficacy than needling with no stimulus. Even if a practitioner is employing a non-needle modality in the treatment, it will be more effective if that modality produces a sensation of some sort akin to the Qi sensation. This sensation varies from point to point and from patient to patient. In general, patients variously describe it as feeling like a deep ache, a tightness, a numbness, an electrical feeling, or several other sensations that stand quite apart from a simple needle-stick feeling. If a practitioner is approaching this book with a background of non-Qi sensation needling technique, we suggest they seek tutelage from a practitioner who is skilled in this method, and to take it easy with their patients until they gain experience with this method. The difference between eliciting a good and effective Qi sensation in a patient and sending them through the roof is often a matter of very finely tuned needle technique. This can only be acquired from expert guidance and careful practice. If this is your situation, please be patient with yourself and realize that it takes time and experience to needle for the Qi sensation at all the points safely and effectively.

Symptom Aggravation: In approximately ten to twenty percent of cases treated with our distal method, an aggravation of the symptom will occur within the first 24 hours following a treatment. This is almost always a good sign, and this should be conveyed to the patient. Usually a symptom aggravation will last 24 to 48 hours; when it subsides, a significant degree of the original symptom will diminish with it. Aggravations as such constitute a kind of "breakthrough" phenomena and seldom occur more than once or twice with any given patient. We make it a policy in our own practices to inform our new patients about this possibility in advance of their first treatment.

More Than Pain Relief: It should also be emphasized to the patient that the use of these points accomplishes more than simple pain relief. Numbness can be treated effectively with the proper corresponding points as well, and overall circulation in the area being distally treated is also improved. Increased circulation can speed healing time.

Case Studies: Once again, please take the time to read through all of the case studies for the point(s) you are looking up. We have arranged the case studies according to the area of the body being treated, starting with the head and working down to the feet. There is valuable additional information contained within the case studies which may prove relevant to the case you are treating. As in the case with *Twelve and Twelve*, we are very interested in hearing from our readers. We welcome any questions, comments, or criticisms, and realize that it is through these encounters that everyone discovers new opportunities for learning and growth.

Chapter 3
Acupuncture Points

Location, Common Indications And Special Applications

(The "Special Applications" sections for each point have been discovered through painstaking research and many hours of clinical testing by the authors)

❖ **Small Intestine 3** (Houxi)

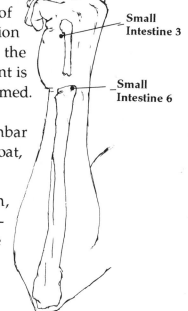

LOCATION: On the lateral or ulnar side of the hand, the point is located at the junction of the red and white skin, proximal to the fifth metacarpophalyngeal joint. The point is on the crease made when a loose fist is formed. (See Figure 1.)

COMMON INDICATIONS: Neck pain, lumbar pain, pain in shoulder and elbow, sore throat, night sweating, fever.

◆ SPECIAL APPLICATION: Neck pain, especially Tai Yang type (generally aggravated by flexion and extension of the neck). For one-sided headache needle the same side, for neck pain either side ah shi point. See case studies pages 50, 53.

Small Intestine 3

Small Intestine 6

Figure 1

❖ Small Intestine 6 (Yanglao)

LOCATION: In the bony cleft found on the radial side of the styloid process of the ulna. This point is best located with the palm resting on the chest. (See Figure 1.)

COMMON INDICATIONS: Pain in the shoulder, elbow and arm, blurred vision.

◆ SPECIAL APPLICATIONS: Scapular pain, pain between medial border of scapula and spine. Needle the same side as the pain. See case studies pages 75, 78.

❖ Large Intestine 5 (Yangxi)

LOCATION: In the "anatomical snuffbox" formed on the radial side of the dorsum of the wrist, when the thumb is raised, causing the tendons of m. extensor pollicis longus and brevis to stand out. (See Figure 2.)

COMMON INDICATIONS: Headache, wrist pain, toothache.

◆ SPECIAL APPLICATIONS: Sprained or painful ankle. Needle contralateral to the painful side. See case studies pages 121, 124.

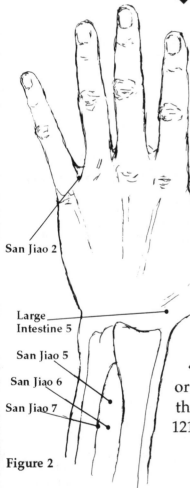

San Jiao 2

Large Intestine 5

San Jiao 5

San Jiao 6

San Jiao 7

Figure 2

❖ San Jiao 2 (Yemen)

LOCATION: In the depression between the metacarpophalyngeal joints of the fourth and fifth fingers, proximal to the web margin. (See Figure 2.)
COMMON INDICATIONS: Headache, sore throat, red eyes, pain in the arm, deafness.

◆ SPECIAL APPLICATION: Sore throat, especially in summer season. Needle either side, but needle the same side if the pain is one-sided. See case studies pages 46, 48.

❖ San Jiao 5 (Waiguan)

LOCATION: Two cun proximal to the wrist crease, in the depression between the radius and the ulna. (Note: the distance from the wrist to the elbow crease is twelve cun.) (See Figure 2.)
COMMON INDICATIONS: Fever, headache, deafness, neck pain, rib pain, constipation.

◆ SPECIAL APPLICATIONS: Constipation, rib pain. Either side, or test for ah shi point to determine which side to needle for pain. See case studies pages 91, 93, 95, 104.

Lung 6

❖ San Jiao 6 (Zhigou)

LOCATION: Three cun proximal to the wrist crease, one cun above San Jiao 5. (See Figure 2.)
COMMON INDICATIONS: Fever, rib pain, deafness, vomiting, pain in shoulder and arm.

Figure 3

◆ **SPECIAL APPLICATIONS**: Constipation, rib pain. Needle the contralateral side for rib pain. See case studies pages 91, 93, 104.

❖ San Jiao 7 (Huizong)

LOCATION: Three cun above the wrist, lateral to San Jiao 6, on the radial side of the ulna, between SJ6 and the ulna. (See Figure 2.)

COMMON INDICATIONS: Ear pain, arm pain, deafness.

◆ **SPECIAL APPLICATIONS**: Constipation, rib pain. Needle the contralateral side for rib pain. See case study page 95.

❖ Lung 6 (Kongzui)

LOCATION: The distance from the inside wrist crease to the inside elbow crease measures as twelve cun. Locating the midpoint on the palmar aspect of the forearm, the point is in a sensitive depression approximately seven cun up from the wrist, on the radial side. (See Figure 3.)

COMMON INDICATIONS: Cough, hemoptysis, pain in chest, hemorrhoids.

◆ **SPECIAL APPLICATIONS**: Upper lumbar or lower thoracic pain. Needle or bleed contralateral to the pain. See case study page 111.

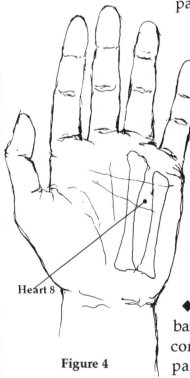

Heart 8

Figure 4

❖ Heart 8 (Shaofu)

LOCATION: On the palm, between the fourth and fifth metacarpal bones. The point is where the tip of the little finger touches when the hand is made into a fist. (See Figure 4.)
COMMON INDICATIONS: Palpitations, pain in little finger, urinary problems.

◆ SPECIAL APPLICATION: Headache (migraine type). Needle contralateral to the pain. See case studies pages 22, 24.

❖ Lung 2a (Yunmen)

LOCATION: Find the depression located just below the acromial extremity of the clavicle. This point is Lung 2. Lung 2a can be located wherever there is a sensitive spot in this vicinity, it is often slightly lateral to Lung 2 on the deltoid muscle. (See Figure 5.)

COMMON INDICATIONS: Cough, asthma, pain in the chest, shoulder or arm. (See Figure 5.)

◆ SPECIAL APPLICATION: Ankle pain or sprain. Needle contralateral to the pain. See case study page 119.

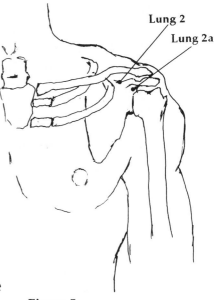

Lung 2

Lung 2a

Figure 5

❖ Spleen 9 (Yinlingquan)

LOCATION: In the depression below the medial epicondyle of the tibia, in the sensitive spot. (See Figure 6.)
COMMON INDICATIONS: Abdominal pain, diarrhea, jaundice, edema, pain in the knee.

◆ SPECIAL APPLICATION: Headache, frontal type. Needle either side, test for ah shi point to determine which side to use. See case studies pages 34, 37.

❖ Spleen 9a

LOCATION: On the sensitive spot, usually one to two cun below SP9. (See Figure 6.)

◆ SPECIAL APPLICATION: Shoulder pain. (Lateral deltoid or Shao Yang area). Needle contralateral to the pain. See case study page 61.

❖ Spleen 7 (Lougu)

LOCATION: The distance from SP9 to the tip of the medial malleolus measures as thirteen cun. SP7 is located on this line, posterior to the tibia, about six cun above the medial malleolus. (See Figure 6.)
COMMON INDICATIONS: Abdominal pain and distention, pain or problems with the knee and leg.

◆ SPECIAL APPLICATION: Menopausal problems. Needle either side, test for ah shi point to determine which side to use. See case studies pages 106, 108.

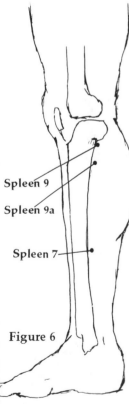

Spleen 9

Spleen 9a

Spleen 7

Figure 6

❖ Kidney 3 (Taixi)

LOCATION: In the depression between the medial malleolus and the achilles tendon, level with the tip of the medial malleolus. (See Figure 6.)

COMMON INDICATIONS: Sore throat, insomnia, tinnitus, nocturnal emission, impotence, low back pain.

◆ SPECIAL APPLICATION: Low back pain. (sacroiliac joint area.) Needle contralateral to the pain. See case studies pages 115, 117.

❖ Stomach 32 (Futu)

LOCATION: In the sensitive spot approximately six cun above the lateral superior border of the patella. (See Figure 7.)

COMMON INDICATIONS: Problems with the lower extremities, lumbar and iliac pain.

◆ SPECIAL APPLICATIONS: Chest pain, heartburn. Needle either side. See case study page 85.

❖ Stomach 36 (Zusanli)

LOCATION: About three cun, or four fingers' distance below the knee approximately one fingers' breadth lateral from the tibia. (See Figure 7.)

COMMON INDICATIONS: Pain in the lower leg/ knee, digestive, heart, and low immune function.

◆ SPECIAL APPLICATION: Pain due to hiatal hernia. Needle either side, or test for ah shi point to determine which side to use. See case studies pages 87, 89.

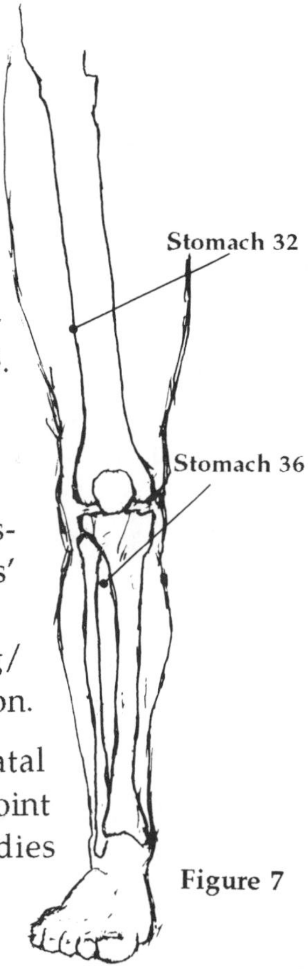

Stomach 32

Stomach 36

Figure 7

❖ Stomach 41 (Jiexi)

LOCATION: On the dorsum of the ankle in the depression between the tendons of m. extensor digitorum longus and hallucis longus. (See Figure 8.)

COMMON INDICATIONS: Pain in the ankle and foot, headache, abdominal distention constipation.

◆ SPECIAL APPLICATIONS: Shoulder pain, (frontal, or Yang Ming area) carpal tunnel or wrist pain (palmar aspect of wrist). Needle on same side. See case studies pages 59, 64, 73.

❖ Gall Bladder 30 (Huantiao)

LOCATION: Draw a line from the prominence of the greater trochanter to the hiatus of the sacrum, marking the distance off in one third increments. GB30 is located at the most lateral of the three marks. (See Figure 9.)

COMMON INDICATIONS: Problems with the lower back hip, and leg.

◆ SPECIAL APPLICATION: Shoulder pain in the trapezius area. (GB21 and SJ15 area.) Needle contralateral to the pain. See case studies pages 55, 57.

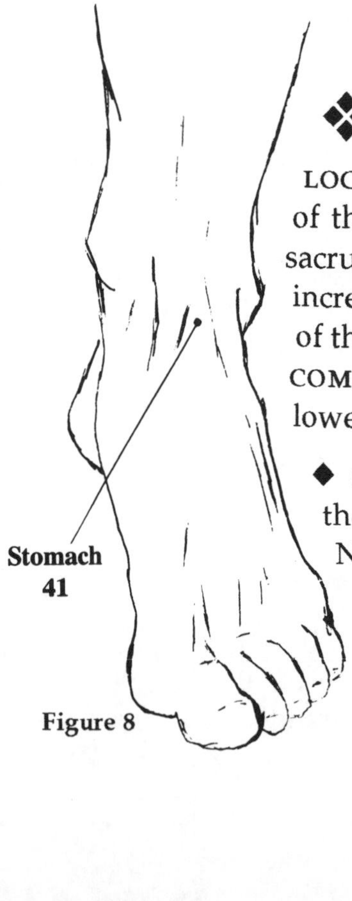

Stomach 41

Figure 8

Gall Bladder 31 (Fengshi)

LOCATION: On the midline of the lateral thigh, the point is in the sensitive spot, approximately where the tip of the middle finger reaches when the straightened arm is held close to the side. (See Figure 9.)

COMMON INDICATIONS: Pain and other problems with the lower leg.

◆ **SPECIAL APPLICATION**: One-sided headache. Needle either side, test for ah shi point to determine which side to use. See case studies pages 28, 31, 32.

 Gall Bladder 32 (Zhongdu)

LOCATION: In the sensitive spot on the midline of the lateral thigh, approximately two cun below GB31. (The distance from the greater trochanter to the epicondyle of the femur is measured as 19 cun. If you prefer measuring, GB31 and 32 are respectively located at 7 and 5 cun above the epicondyle of the femur). (See Figure 9.)

COMMON INDICATIONS: Pain and other problems of thigh, knee, lower leg.

◆ **SPECIAL APPLICATION**: TMJ pain. Needle either side, test for ah shi point to determine which side to use. See case studies pages 39, 42.

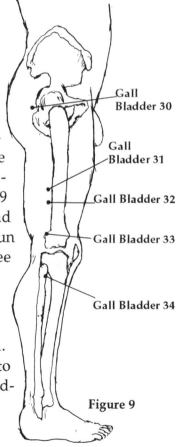

Gall
Bladder 30

Gall
Bladder 31

Gall Bladder 32

Gall Bladder 33

Gall Bladder 34

Figure 9

❖ Gall Bladder 33 (Xiyanguan)

LOCATION: In the depression lateral to the knee joint, between the tendon of biceps femoris and the femur. (See Figure 9.)
COMMON INDICATIONS: Problems with the knee and lower leg.

◆ SPECIAL APPLICATIONS: Elbow pain or tennis elbow. Needle contralateral to the pain. See case studies pages 67, 69.

❖ Gall Bladder 34 (Yanglingquan)

LOCATION: on the lateral aspect of the lower leg, in the depression distal and anterior to the head of the fibula. (See Figure 9.)

COMMON INDICATIONS: Problems with the lower extremities, jaundice, pain in hypochondriac region, vomiting.

◆ SPECIAL APPLICATION: Rib pain (Needle contralaterally). Lower abdominal pain (Needle the same side). See case studies pages 98, 100, 102.

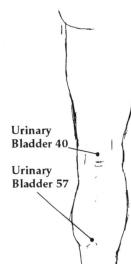

Urinary Bladder 40

Urinary Bladder 57

❖ Urinary Bladder 40 (Weizhong)

LOCATION: In the center of the popliteal fossa. (See Figure 10.)
COMMON INDICATIONS: Problems with the lower extremities, low back pain.

◆ SPECIAL APPLICATION: Low back pain, hemorrhoids. Treat either or both sides with bleeding technique, check for prominent capillaries. See case study page 113.

Figure 10

Urinary Bladder 57 (Chengshan)

LOCATION: At about the midpoint of the posterior aspect of the lower leg, on the midline drawn from UB40 to the Achilles tendon at the ankle. The point is found in the center of the belly of m. gastrocnemius. (See Figure 10.)

COMMON INDICATIONS: Low back pain, lower leg pain, hemorrhoids.

◆ SPECIAL APPLICATION: Upper back pain (bleeding and needle). Needle or bleed contralateral to the pain. See case studies pages 81, 83.

Chapter 4

Case Studies

———◆•◆•◆———

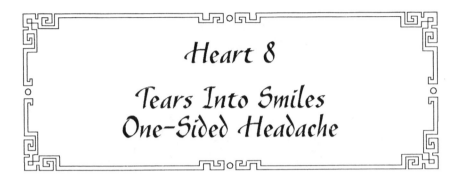

Heart 8

Tears Into Smiles
One-Sided Headache

Female, Age 29

This patient was a headache sufferer who was referred to Dr. Tan by one of her office co-workers. She had been suffering from one-sided headaches intermittently for many years. She called his office at about four o'clock one afternoon when she felt one of her headaches coming on. Dr. Tan was able to squeeze her into the busy schedule, in spite of the fact that this was her first treatment, and there were the usual forms and paperwork to be completed. It was obvious that she was suffering, and Dr. Tan convinced her that it was perfectly fine she was there, as long as she didn't mind waiting a few minutes. She was the last patient of the day, and by the time she was ushered into the treatment room she was in so much pain that she could not keep herself from crying.

She described the onset of the headache as beginning in the area around Gall Bladder 1, then progressing along the side of her head, following the Gall Bladder channel, and down to the base of her neck. The pain was on the left side of her head. Her pulse was excess (shi) and wiry; her tongue exhibited a red tip.

22

Upon questioning, she explained that the previous night she had stayed up very late, ingested several drinks, and only gotten about 2 hours sleep before reporting to work the next morning. She recalled that lack of sleep often preceded one of her headaches.

The only needle used for this treatment was inserted at Heart 8 on the right or contralateral side. The needle was stimulated by twirling continuously for 1 minute, at which time the patient claimed the pain in her head had subsided completely. She was still experiencing a pressure-like sensation in the area around her eye, so the needle was left in place and stimulated in the same fashion for approximately 30 seconds about every 15 minutes. After about 1 hour the pressure sensation and all of the pain were gone. Having arrived in tears, this patient left smiling, glad that she had listened to her co-worker and taken a chance on acupuncture.

Summary

This case, while being quite simple and dramatic in nature, is actually not very unusual in Dr. Tan's clinic. The patient, impressed by the effect of her treatment, became a regular patient, and eventually her headaches were a thing of the past.

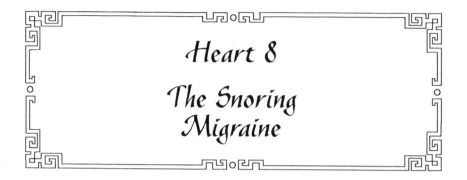

Heart 8

The Snoring Migraine

Female, Age 65

Originally having sought treatment from Dr. Tan for low-back pain, this patient had also mentioned her occasional migraine attacks. (For more information on low-back pain treatment, please see the section on the "Ling Ku Combination" in our first book, *Twelve and Twelve in Acupuncture*.) Once her back pain had been cleared up, her headaches became a source of increasing concern and bother to her.

She had been suffering from intermittent severe headaches for at least 5 years. The headaches were always one-sided and would typically begin behind the eye and radiate to the side or the top of the head. The pain would reach an intensity severe enough to cause nausea and vomiting in many cases, often forcing her to bedrest until the pain ran its course. Conventional prescription and over-the-counter drugs afforded little or no relief from such a relentless headache.

When one of her headaches began, it would gain in intensity until a peak level of pain was reached after about 6 to 8 hours.

Once established, the headache could last for 24 hours or longer.

At the outset of the series of treatments she was to receive for her headache problem, Dr. Tan instructed her to wait until she could actually feel a headache coming on, and then to call the office or just come in to be treated. There are many possible ways in which this type of headache problem might be treated. The key lies in the practitioner's ability to properly diagnose the channels involved and to identify any underlying internal imbalances which may be contributing to their cause. An excellent way to test a theoretical diagnosis is to try a treatment based upon it when the symptom—in this case pain—is actually present. In this way we can receive the best and most relevant feedback possible on the accuracy of our hypothesis. And since Traditional Chinese Medicine typically makes little or no use of objective lab tests, this type of practical objectivity is a very sensible course of action.

It wasn't long before she began to feel a headache building; following the doctor's instructions, she came straight into the office one afternoon. The headache was on the right side of her head and had been intensifying for about 3 hours by the time of her treatment. In other words, she was suffering from a significant degree of pain at this time. Her pulses were wiry and tight, and her tongue had purplish edges.

For treatment, Dr. Tan needled Heart 8 and Gall Bladder 41 on the left, San Jiao 3 and Liver 3 on the right. The principal point in this treatment, H8, was needled contralateral to the pain. After obtaining a substantial Qi sensation on all four needles, the patient began to feel the pain subside about 1 minute into the treatment. The needles were left in place for 1 hour and were stimulated every 15 minutes. At the conclusion of the treatment, the headache was completely gone.

This point selection was employed as the core treatment strategy for her subsequent treatments, which were administered as needed (when she had a headache during Dr. Tan's office hours). Over the following 6 months, she received fifteen treatments.

During this time, Dr. Tan discovered an interesting pattern. He found that her husband, who snored in his sleep, would periodically snore more loudly than usual. It seemed that the headaches would recur not long after one of these intense snoring episodes began. The doctor suggested that his patient and her husband try sleeping in separate rooms during these times. The husband agreed to try it, although he seemed a little resentful at what he probably viewed as an intrusion into their personal lives. However, after trying this arrangement for a while, the patient's headaches ceased to recur as quickly after treatment, and the husband grudgingly admitted that Dr. Tan probably was right. After seeing this trend hold up consistently for over a month, he even thanked the doctor, because his wife's overall disposition had improved so much! To date, the patient still suffers occasional headaches, but they are much less severe and short-lived in nature.

Summary

Two important points that Dr. Tan feels need to be emphasized are illustrated in this case. First, the positive results from the treatment can confirm a diagnosis. Second, to discern whether or not a symptom's recurrence following an apparently successful treatment, is due to a flaw in the treatment plan, or to an aggravation caused by the patient's lifestyle or environment. Of course, we should always cast a critical eye upon our practice of medicine, but that criticism should be tempered by a thorough examination of all possible complications. Don't give up on a treatment strategy that yields good results until you are certain there are no underlying aggravating factors present.

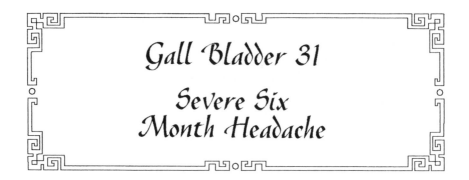

Gall Bladder 31

Severe Six
Month Headache

Female, Age 30

This patient had been suffering from severe headache symptoms for at least 6 months. She had been diagnosed as suffering from migraine headaches by an M.D. who prescribed appropriate medications. The medications not only failed to improve her headache symptoms but generated side-effects which affected her digestion and sleep. The headaches occurred on an almost daily basis. They were always on the left side of her head, affecting both the temporal region and the area behind her left eye.

Gall Bladder 31 was needled on the right side, with Liver 3 selected on the left for balance. She reported a significant lessening of the pain after about 5 minutes of treatment time. The needles were stimulated at 5 to 10 minute intervals for the remainder of the treatment, which lasted about 40 minutes. At that time she reported no detectable headache symptoms and remained symptom-free for over 48 hours. Headache symptoms began to recur 3 days after her first treatment, at which time she was treated again.

She was treated in this manner twice a week for three weeks; it was then suspected that the type of birth control medication she was using might be contributing to the headache's recurrence. This conjecture was based on the observation that the headaches' intensity seemed to increase at a specific point in the patient's menstrual cycle. Dr. Tan asked the patient to consult with her physician about the possibility of changing her prescription. The prescription was changed, but no immediate improvement was noticed. As she continued to receive acupuncture treatment on the twice-weekly basis, the frequency of the headaches began to diminish. After her eleventh acupuncture treatment, she no longer suffered from headache symptoms between appointments. In all, she received a total of nineteen treatments and reported no headache symptoms 8 months after her course of treatment was concluded.

Summary

The points used in her treatment varied from time to time, but Gall Bladder 31 was always used to directly address the headache symptoms.

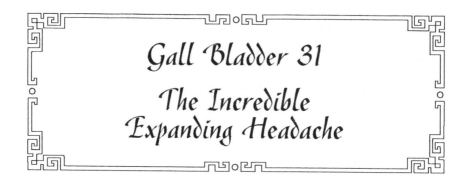

Gall Bladder 31
The Incredible
Expanding Headache

Female, Age 32

This particular woman had been suffering for 2 to 3 years from chronic headache symptoms which usually occurred on the left side of her head, expanding to affect the whole head as the headache worsened. Their frequency averaged two to three times a week.

At the time of her first treatment, her headache was in the early one-sided stage. She was nauseous and she a wiry pulse. Since the majority of her pain was in the vicinity of the left temple, Gall Bladder 31 on the right side was needled. The patient expressed an extreme fear of needles, coming for acupuncture treatment only out of a sense of desperation. For this reason, only GB31 was needled, but the effect of that one needle was quite dramatic, eliminating the headache entirely within 5 minutes.

After the headache was gone, her pulse was checked again and found to have changed from a wiry, excess condition to a sinking deep one, especially so in the Kidney position. It was determined that a Kidney deficiency constitution was the major underlying factor in this case, and a strategy to tonify involving herbs as well as acupuncture, was devised. The patient's confidence in acupuncture was greatly enhanced by the success of her introductory treatment, and she was easily persuaded to allow the addition of some extra needles for the purpose of improving her health.

In all, she received a total of twenty treatments at intervals of twice a week at first, reducing to weekly treatments as her condition stabilized. GB31 was used in the first fifteen treatments and was discontinued for the final five due to no recurrence of headache symptoms for approximately 3 weeks.

Summary

This case was of special interest due to the severity of her pain symptoms which caused a change in the fundamental nature of her pulse, completely masking the underlying deficiency signs. Here, the fast-acting effect of GB31 enabled a more accurate diagnosis to be achieved.

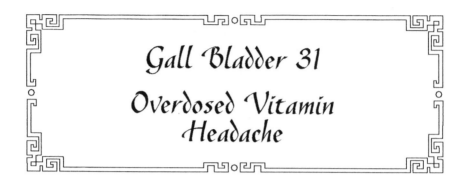

Gall Bladder 31

Overdosed Vitamin Headache

Male, Age 37

This is a one treatment case for a severe one-sided headache which may have been induced by an overdose of a vasodilating mineral supplement. The patient had, for stress-relief purposes, ingested 1,000 mg. of both potassium and magnesium in their highly absorbable orotate form. This induced a rapid vasodilating effect which apparently produced the symptoms of a severe migraine-like headache. The patient normally experienced no headaches at all.

He described the headache as being centered at the left temple, extending into the left eye with an intensity that he described as "blinding." His pulse was wiry; his blood pressure was 110/70. Gall Bladder 31 on the right side was needled, producing a strong Qi sensation. Within 5 minutes the headache symptoms began to subside; at the conclusion of the treatment 45 minutes later, he experienced more than a 50 percent reduction of the symptoms. He later reported that the remainder of his headache disappeared while he was being driven home from his treatment. There was no recurrence.

Summary

A one-sided headache, even one due to a nutrient overdose, can often be treated with GB31. Palpation of this point on the leg contralateral to the headache should find it very sensitive.

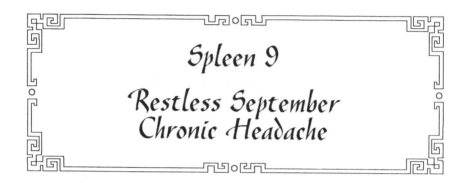

Spleen 9

Restless September
Chronic Headache

Female, Age 32

This patient came in for treatment complaining of chronic headaches which had been bothering her for years. The headaches always seemed to be worse in the summer months, especially between July and September. The headache was invariably a frontal one, extending across both sides of her forehead.

Upon examination, her pulse was thin and deficient, especially in the guan (middle) position. Her tongue was slightly pale, with toothmarks and a purplish tinge along its edges. She also stated that she had difficulty getting enough sleep during the summer, when excessive activity, or just plain restlessness would often prevent her from getting adequate rest.

Upon palpation, both Spleen 9 points were extremely sensitive to moderate pressure.

For treatment, SP9 was needled bilaterally. Large Intestine 4 was also needled bilaterally for its Qi regulating effect, especially

34

upon the region of the face and forehead. A good Qi sensation was obtained with all four needles. The needles were stimulated at 15 minute intervals, and the treatment lasted about an hour, at which time she could detect about a 50 percent improvement.

This improvement largely held up until the time of her second appointment later that week. The same points were again needled in the same fashion (as they would be for the entire course of her treatment). By the conclusion of treatment number two, she reported feeling an additional 20 percent improvement, and most of this gain maintained itself until the time of her third treatment, early in the following week.

At the time of her third appointment, she reported that although the degree of pain and the frequency of her headaches had both shown a significant improvement, she was still having as much trouble with her sleep habits as ever. For this treatment, the point Yin Tang was added, as well as an ear tack in the auricular Shen Men. Her sleep was much better that night, and in future treatments an ear Shen Men would prove sufficient on the occasions when she again experienced some sleep problems.

She continued to be treated in this way twice a week, with more or less steady improvements in terms of less frequent and severe headaches. By the occasion of her twenty-fifth treatment, no headache symptoms were recurring. She was treated another seven times to consolidate the effect. To date, she reports no further problems in this area, and is also sleeping much better.

Summary

Often in summer, due to the energetic nature of the season, people do not get enough sleep. Yet in spite of their feelings of abundant energy, they still can get run down at this time of year if they don't get proper rest and nutrition. We have found that chronic headaches tend to get worse in summer time are often a clear indication that the patient is not getting enough sleep. Correcting this will go a long way towards solving their headache problems.

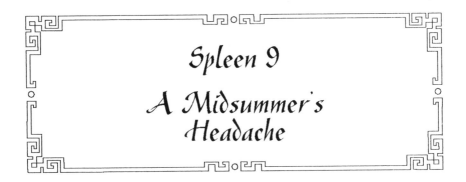

Spleen 9

A Midsummer's Headache

A forty-year-old woman had been suffering from a continual headache for 1 week. She was somewhat overweight. She described the pain as being located on both sides as well as in the center (glabella) of her forehead. The pain was heavy-feeling and constant. Her pulse was bounding and slippery. Her tongue did not exhibit any remarkable characteristics, appearing relatively normal upon inspection. The season was the middle of summer.

For treatment, Spleen 9 was needled bilaterally. Strong stimulus was given to the needles continuously for 2 to 3 minutes, after which the lights were turned out in the treatment room, and she was left alone to rest. When checked upon 15 minutes later, she said that the headache was noticeably better. The needles were again stimulated for approximately 30 seconds to 1 minute, followed with another 15 minutes' rest.

This process was repeated three more times, for a total treatment time of $1\frac{1}{2}$ hours. The only two points needled were Spleen 9 bilaterally.

At the conclusion of the treatment she reported feeling no detectable headache symptoms. There was no recurrence.

Summary

This is a simple case that illustrates the potential effectiveness of the point SP9 in treatment of frontal headache, especially in summer time. Exactly why certain points have a stronger effect in certain seasons is an intriguing subject, one that we intend to address in an upcoming publication.

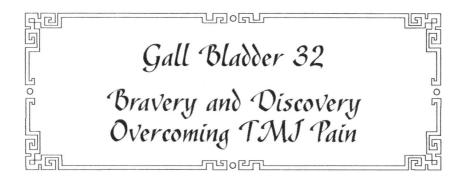

Gall Bladder 32
Bravery and Discovery
Overcoming TMJ Pain

A thirty-year-old woman who had been diagnosed with TMJ (temporal-mandibular joint) syndrome was referred to the clinic for acupuncture treatment. She appeared to be very nervous and confessed that she was somewhat terrified at the prospect of having needles inserted into her body. But the pain of her condition had driven her to overcome her fear in the hope of obtaining relief. She was especially frightened at the prospect of having needles inserted into her face and jaw area, so we decided that she would need to be treated with an entirely distal method.

Upon examination, she was found to be unable to open her mouth wide enough to fit two of her fingers into it. Her pulse was wiry and tight. She reported the pain as being bad enough at times that it caused migraine-like headaches which could persist for hours.

For the first treatment, the points San Jiao 3 and Gall Bladder 41 were needled bilaterally, since her TMJ problem presented itself on both sides of her jaw. A strong Qi sensation, in consideration of her anxiety, was not elicited. Instead, SJ3 was connected to GB41 on each side with an electrical stimulator to provide a continual stimulus to her system. In general, we do not feel that electrical stimulation is as effective as a surrogate for the true Qi sensation. But in situations like this one, it has its place.

By the end of her treatment she had relaxed considerably, and the headache she had come in with was gone. After this first treatment, she was only able to open her jaw a little wider than before. She received two treatments per week. Treatments two and three were given using the same points and stimulation, with approximately 30 percent improvement in her jaw range of motion and in pain relief. Since we were employing a very gentle approach with this patient, the response generated was satisfactory enough to warrant continuing treatment in this fashion.

However, at the time of her fourth treatment the patient informed us that the hand and foot points had become too painful for her, so another plan had to be devised. Since we had often used Gall Bladder 31 to treat headaches, it seemed reasonable to palpate that area on her to check for ah shi sensitivity. GB31 was not very sensitive itself, but GB32 and two ah shi points just below it on the Gall Bladder line were all very tender to the touch. Since the patient did not have any objection, these three points were needled bilaterally. Following this treatment plan, the patient was able to gradually increase the degree to which she could open her mouth without discomfort. By the eighth treatment she was able to fit three of her fingers in her mouth without any problem. By adding the ear point Shen Men into the treatment, the patient found it easier to tolerate a stronger Qi sensation, and progress in her case was quickened. In all, the patient received a total of twenty-three treatments in this case, with twenty of them being comprised of the GB32 group of points. She was under treatment for about 12 weeks in all. At that time, she was able to consistently open her mouth to three fingers' width with no problem and reported no recurrence of her headaches and other TMJ-related pains.

Summary

Some acupuncturists may view a patient with an unusually great fear of needles as something less than a blessing . . . but such people are braving, in most cases, a tremendous phobia. This constitutes a small triumph of the human spirit—it presents a valuable opportunity to observe an individual grow in a positive way. A special thanks is owed to this patient, because it is through the special challenge that she posed to us with her case, that we were able to discover a valuable new clinical application.

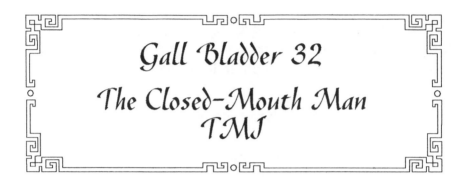

Gall Bladder 32
The Closed-Mouth Man
TMJ

A thirty-five-year-old man with a high-stress job came in for treatment of his painful TMJ (temporal-mandibular joint) condition. Job stress would often aggravate the symptoms, which included difficulty in opening the mouth, headache, clicking, and especially constant pain in the joint area. He occasionally would be unable to sleep due to the pain. TMJ had been diagnosed as the problem by both his dentist and an M.D. To treat the condition he had been given a special dental splint designed to correct his bite and TMJ function, with instructions to wear it in his mouth more or less constantly. The splint did help to reduce the degree of severity in pain, but the feeling of tightness in his jaw seemed unaffected. Also, after several months of wearing the splint, the pain, while less, was still constantly present as a dull ache. He still experienced occasional sharp pain in the area as well, usually once or twice a day, and these sharp pains would often seem to act as a trigger for a temporal headache. It was at this point, after realizing he had reached a plateau in his recovery process, that he came in for an acupuncture consultation.

Upon examination, the masseter muscle on both sides was

found to be very tight and sensitive to palpation. The temporalis muscle was also very tight and sensitive to the touch. When asked to try opening his mouth as wide as he could, he could barely open wide enough to insert two of his fingers. His pulse was tight and bouncy. Upon further palpation, the Gall Bladder 32 area was found to be very sensitive; that point and an ah shi point between GB32 and 33 were the most reactive.

For treatment, GB32 and the ah shi points were needled bilaterally, since both sides of his jaw were affected. While these points were stimulated, he was asked to open and close his mouth; he found that he was immediately able to open it further, with less pain. At this point, he was able to insert three of his fingers into his mouth with only a slight discomfort. However, after being left alone for a few minutes, the stiffness in the jaw muscles returned. Although it disappeared again when the needles were re-stimulated, it seemed as if the response was not lasting very long. At this time, two local points were inserted on each side, GB6 and Stomach 6. GB6 was inserted horizontally with the needle threaded posteriorly towards GB8, about 1.5 cun. ST6 was needled perpendicularly. An electric stimulator set at 2 cps. was applied, connecting the GB6 points together and the Stomach channel points together.

These points were left in place with the stimulator attached for about 30 minutes more. During this time, the distal Gall Bladder points were stimulated four more times at intervals ranging from 5 to 10 minutes apart. Before the end of the treatment, but after the local points were removed, the distal points were stimulated one last time with the patient instructed to try opening and closing his mouth. At this time, he was able to insert three fingers into his mouth with no pain or tension at all, a result that seemed to hold up after the needles were removed.

For the next 8 weeks he was treated with this method, twice weekly.

During the first 2 to 3 weeks, the symptoms would reassert themselves between treatments. But overall, the degree of severity was becoming consistently less. During these first few weeks he also continued to wear his prescribed splint constantly. After the third week of treatment, he reported a significant change. The symptoms had ceased to recur, with slight stiffness, clicking, and a dull ache manifesting after high stress. After the fourth week of treatment, he decided to try going for extended periods of time without the splint, experiencing no symptoms of aggravation. After the sixth week of acupuncture treatment, his improvement was so great that one day he forgot to wear the splint altogether, even when he went to bed. The next day he felt no aggravation from this lapse at all. The only symptom persisting at this time was the click, which would result on occasion when he opened his mouth widely. By week eight in his treatment the frequency of his office visits was reduced to once a week for 4 more weeks; from then on treatment was given only on an as-needed basis.

Four months later, he returned to the office to get an herbal formula for some cold and flu symptoms; at that time he reported experiencing no TMJ symptoms at all.

Summary

TMJ syndrome can often be difficult to treat, either with western or Oriental medicine. This is especially true for severe cases of TMJ. Here, it was necessary to add strong local treatment to the overall treatment strategy. This combined approach yielded the desired results.

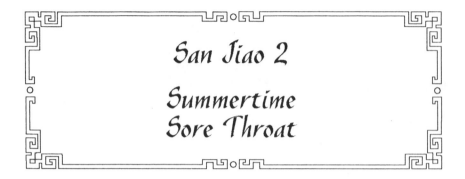

San Jiao 2

Summertime
Sore Throat

A thirty-one-year-old man had been diagnosed as suffering from Candida syndrome for about 5 years. The main symptoms of this condition—fatigue, digestive problems, abdominal bloating, and diarrhea—had manifested themselves after an extremely heavy course of antibiotic therapy; they had been bothering him ever since. He was referred for acupuncture treatment by a massage therapist, mainly for help with his constant abdominal pain and distention.

After 3 weeks of treatment, the diarrhea had stopped completely, and after four weeks the abdominal bloating and pain were gone as well. His fatigue symptoms had only improved slightly at this time. He was also being troubled by a sore throat that he seemed to wake up with every morning, especially during the current season, which was summer. The pain in his throat would persist for about 5 hours after he woke up, gradually fading as the day progressed. His pulse was wiry and slippery, and his tongue had red edges with toothmarks. The decision was made at this point to focus the acupuncture treatment on his sore throat and fatigue symptoms.

For treatment, the principal point selected was San Jiao 2, with Lung 10 chosen to assist and balance it. The points were needled bilaterally, since the sore throat symptoms was on both sides. On the leg, Stomach 36 and Spleen 9 were needled to help build his Qi and to provide a balanced treatment. At the conclusion of the first treatment of this series, he reported having no sore throat sensation at all. The symptoms of fatigue and sore throat were gone for 2 days, then began to return. This effect, although not permanent, was considered a good sign, indicating that the treatment strategy was on the right track. Treatment was continued with this group of points on a twice-weekly basis for 12 weeks. At this time his sore throat and fatigue symptoms had not returned for 3 weeks. After week twelve, regular treatments were discontinued, though he continues to come in every 4 to 8 weeks for a health maintenance treatment.

Summary

Some practitioners may be aware of the indication of SJ2 for sore throat treatment, but considering the effectiveness we have observed, we feel that it is greatly underutilized. It is made even more effective by the addition of LU10. Additionally, we find that it seems to work the most powerfully for sore throat treatment in the summer time.

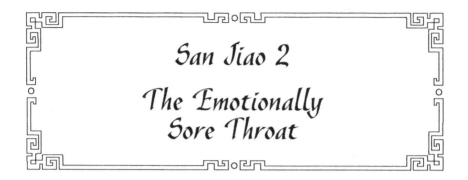

San Jiao 2

The Emotionally Sore Throat

A twenty-nine-year-old man, an author and artist, had returned from a weekend personal growth seminar. Several exercises designed to facilitate the release of suppressed feelings were practiced at the seminar. Many of these exercises involved screaming, and the patient, while feeling better emotionally, came home with a sore throat which was audibly raspy and hoarse. His pulse was somewhat wiry and deficient, and his tongue had a reddish tip and a thin white coat. He had also quit smoking, one pack per day, just the week before.

For treatment, the principle point used was San Jiao 2, with Lung 10 added on the opposite side to assist. SJ2 was needled on the left and LU10 on the right. Having acquired the sore throat through a great deal of emotional screaming, a point on the Heart meridian, Heart 5, was also needled on the right to help resettle his spirit. A Ren channel point, Ren 17, was also added as this point is very useful with emotion-related conditions. On the legs, Kidney 6 was needled on the left and Urinary Bladder 62 on the right. These points added more balance to the treatment, with KD6 also helping to moisten the throat, while UB62 helped with the emotions. A few minutes into the treatment, he reported feeling better, and by the end of the treatment, his throat felt completely normal. The treatment lasted about 50 minutes, with the needles being stimulated every 10 minutes. When he left the clinic, his voice was much clearer sounding with only a hint of its former roughness. He was given some mild Loquat Herb Syrup, a Chinese sore throat and cough remedy, to help with any slight residual problem.

Summary

This simple one treatment case demonstrates the effectiveness of using San Jiao 2 for sore throat problems, even when due to circumstances such as overuse of the voice. This patient continues to receive periodic treatment to promote his overall well-being. As such, acupuncture has become an essential part of his healthy new lifestyle.

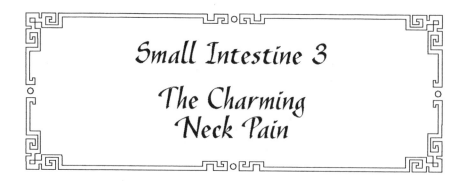

Small Intestine 3

The Charming Neck Pain

This patient came to us with a medical history of psoriasis and rheumatoid arthritis. He was 50 years old and slightly overweight. Most of the arthritis symptoms he had been suffering from were centered in the knees, with some redness and swelling also occurring in his finger joints. His chief complaint and reason for seeing an acupuncturist, however, was neck pain. An M.D. had suspected arthritic involvement in his neck as well and had ordered an MRI. Arthritic changes were not detected, but some disc abnormality between the fifth and sixth cervical was noted. In fact, his M.D. had scheduled him for surgery, giving him about 3 weeks to see if any response could be obtained through acupuncture.

At the time of his first visit, the neck pain had been bothering him for over 2 months. Upon examination, the patient described a constant pain that radiated along the lateral posterior surface of his shoulder and arm down to his elbow. The pain shifted sides, sometimes occurring on the right, sometimes on the left. Palpation of the points Urinary Bladder 10 and Small Intestine 15 bilaterally revealed them to be the most reactive, helping to determine the Tai Yang channels as the ones most involved. The patient was able to rotate his neck laterally with relative ease: flexion and extension, however, were restricted. This finding also pointed towards the Tai Yang channels as being the most affected.

For treatment, we decided to needle bilaterally, since there was no particular side on which the symptom was worse. The points selected were Small Intestine 3 and Urinary Bladder 65. It is worth mentioning that upon bilateral palpation of these points prior to treatment, they displayed an equal degree of sensitivity between left and right, yet another indicator of the need for bilateral treatment. A good Qi sensation was obtained, and the needles were stimulated at approximately 15 minute intervals— the first treatment lasting a bit over 45 minutes. Two days later, at the time of his second treatment, the patient reported minimal improvement, in the neighborhood of 5 to 10 percent. The same points were needled, again bilaterally. Upon returning for his third treatment, the patient again reported only a minimal improvement. A re-examination still showed the Tai Yang area to be the most involved, so once again the same treatment was given. The third time must have been the charm in this case, because after this treatment the patient was happy to report at least 50 percent improvement in the pain and mobility of his neck.

This improvement subsided slightly in the interval between the third and fourth treatments, but was still significant enough to encourage the patient to continue on with the acupuncture. He was treated three times a week during the next 3 weeks. At this time his improvement in pain and mobility was about 80 percent, prompting him to cancel his plans for surgery. He continued to receive treatments twice weekly for 2 more weeks, at which time he was pain-free with no recurrence of his symptoms between treatments.

Summary

Several interesting aspects of this case deserve emphasis. Perhaps most significant is the deviation from our own characteristic style of unilateral needling. Several indicators were presented in this case for such a departure from the usual procedure: (a) the lack of a clearly one-sided presentation of the symptom; (b) the equal sensitivity of the points palpated bilaterally in the region of the pain; and (c) the bilateral sensitivity of the distal points selected for needling.

Also demonstrated in this case is the importance of confidence—on the part of the practitioner—in relation to the diagnosis, as well as the need for the patient to feel confident in the ability of the practitioner. If, after two treatments, we had not been confident in the diagnosis of this case as being primarily a Tai Yang channel problem, we probably would not have gotten the results we obtained by persevering with the treatment strategy. Likewise, if the patient had given up on the acupuncture treatments after two tries, he probably would have submitted to surgery with all of its attendant risks and potential complications. A charming outcome for all involved.

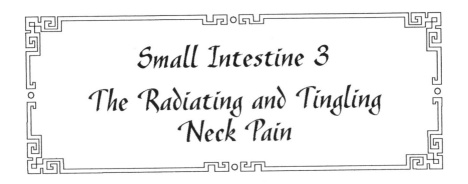

Small Intestine 3
The Radiating and Tingling Neck Pain

A forty-three-year-old woman came in for treatment complaining of neck pain. The pain would occasionally radiate down her right arm to her little finger. Her M.D. had prescribed a muscle relaxer and a non-steroidal anti-inflammatory, both of which had little effect. An orthopedic surgeon had found a likely disc protrusion between the sixth and seventh cervical. He did not recommend surgery at that time, advising her to wait until the problem became more severe. Upon examination, she described the pain as radiating down the lateral or ulnar aspect of her arm, a path coinciding with the Small Intestine channel. Rotation and lateral flexion aggravated the pain. Thus it was decided that the principle channel involved was the Hand-Tai Yang.

For treatment, Small Intestine 3 and Urinary Bladder 65 were chosen bilaterally. Since the patient seemed to be quite nervous and unable to completely relax, a good Qi sensation could not be obtained in this first treatment. This probably accounts for the lack of significant improvement that occurred after this session. By the third treatment she was comfortable enough with the idea of acupuncture that she was able to tolerate a substantial Qi sensation, and at this time she also experienced a good response. After treatment number three, she was treated twice a week for a total of twelve treatments, at which time she was pain-free. The only points used were UB65 and SI3. It was suggested that she return once a week for a while for maintenance treatments to help stabilize the results. However, since her insurance did not cover acupuncture treatment, and she was on a tight budget, she stopped treatment. Her insurance would not pay for acupuncture, which was extremely effective—but it would pay for a surgical procedure, which was not recommended by per physician.

For about 18 months she was fine, at which time tingling in her right arm began to recur. She didn't come in right away for treatment, once again because she would have to pay for treatment with no reimbursement from her insurer. After 2 more months, she the increasing pain forced her in for more treatment. She received two treatments a week for 5 weeks, before the pain was gone again. The pain and tingling recurred again 2 years later, at when she was again treated with the same procedure and frequency. This time it required a total of fourteen treatments to completely resolve, and at the present time there has been no recurrence.

Summary

Treatment in this case was administered bilaterally. Although the radiating pain only occurred on her right side, she generally had pain on both sides of her neck, justifying the bilateral treatment approach. Also worthy of note in this case is yet another example of the necessity of the Qi sensation in order to get a good result.

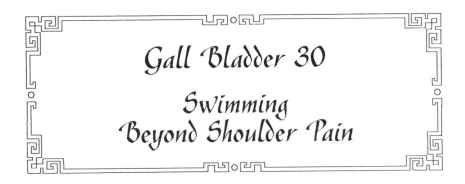

Gall Bladder 30

Swimming
Beyond Shoulder Pain

Female, Age 22

A college athlete, both a swimmer and a rower, came in suffering from extreme sensitivity in her right shoulder. The pain had developed after overtraining for a rowing event. The competition was scheduled in 3 weeks' time, and she wanted to recover as quickly as possible. Aside from this training injury she appeared to be in excellent health.

Both abduction and adduction of her shoulder were severely impaired. Palpation of her affected shoulder revealed the greatest sensitivity and spasm in the region of San Jiao 14, causing her to jump when this point was lightly pressed. Thus it was apparent that the Shao Yang channel was the primary one involved.

For treatment, Gall Bladder 30 on the left side was selected. Although the patient was not a large person, a 2.5 cun needle was used, since the actual Qi field for this point is located quite deep beneath the surface, usually at least 1.5 cun down. (The point itself is quite large in area, about the circumference of a ping pong ball, but the needle must be inserted relatively deep for this point to really be accessed properly.) A strong Qi sensation was obtained, which caused the needle to be grabbed tightly in the tissue. After 5 minutes, the needle was twirled while the patient moved her arm and shoulder in a "swimming" motion. She was amazed to find that her range of motion had increased dramatically in such a short time. The needle was left in place, with the same procedure repeated every 10 minutes for the duration of her treatment. GB30 was the only point used in this one-needle treatment. In addition, an herbal plaster was placed over the injury site.

She was treated in this fashion daily for 5 days. After the first 5 days, she began training again, albeit lightly at first. During the second week following her injury, she received three treatments on an every-other-day basis. She continued to progress, able to train a little more intensely as the days went by. At the end of her third week, she was able to exert herself fully at the oars and was ready for competition.

Summary

This case illustrates the application of acupuncture in the treatment of sports injuries, demonstrating the value of "Sports Acupuncture" for the athlete. In many cases it may not be necessary for an acupuncturist to seek outside help in the treatment of a case such as this one. More specifically, this case points out the necessity of properly needling GB30, in order to obtain the desired result.

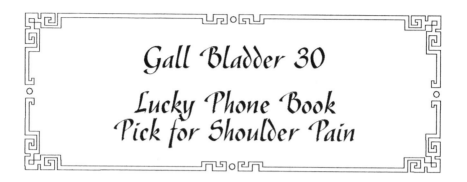

Gall Bladder 30

Lucky Phone Book Pick for Shoulder Pain

A thirty-seven-year-old man, complaining of pain in the trape-zius and related areas of the lateral posterior shoulder, came in for treatment. Having moved to San Diego recently from the Chicago area, he simply picked an acupuncturist out of the phone book . . . fortunately, he picked a very competent one. Back in Chicago, he had received some relief from a practitioner who employed a combination of acupuncture and acupressure massage. Upon examination it became apparent that in addition to the painful trapezius, there was a good deal of sensitivity in the scapular and upper thoracic areas as well. He had a long history of asthma and allergies, clearly aggravated by the change in environment from the humid Midwest to the dry south-western climate.

Also, he exhibited a pronounced scoliosis, clearly a major contributing factor to his upper back and shoulder pain. He described the periodic onset of this pain as a kind of tension, often initiated by stress and/or heavy overhead lifting. The tension slowly progressed into a state so painful that it would interfere with his sleep.

For treatment, the patient was asked to lay face down and to circle his arms in a "swimming" motion, noting the places where he felt the most discomfort and limitation in motion. Then Gall Bladder 30 on the left side was needled and stimulated while the patient moved the right arm around. Not being familiar with this style of acupuncture, he expressed concern as to whether or not we knew what we were doing, but under the given circumstances, he decided to award us the benefit of the doubt.

Happily, within seconds his trust began to pay off, as the range of motion in his right arm and shoulder noticeably increased, accompanied by an immediate decrease in pain and tension on that side. Next, GB30 was needled on the right, the same procedure repeated with the left arm, again with significant results. In addition, two ah shi points were located bilaterally in the trapezius area and needled with electrical stimulation for 15 minutes, leaving the GB30 needles in place. After the local needles were removed, the same procedure was repeated again (i.e., stimulating the left point while moving the right shoulder). At this time, the patient could detect no pain or stiffness at all. Over the following 2 years, he came in periodically for treatment as needed, always with favorable results.

Summary

The pain in this case was due to a longstanding, virtually congenital condition. While the acupuncture was very successful in dealing with the pain, the cause—his lifetime scoliosis—was not affected. However, this is a good case for illustrating the effectiveness of acupuncture as a pain management strategy free from side effects.

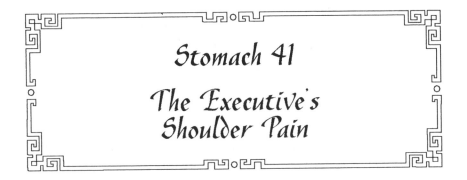

Stomach 41

The Executive's Shoulder Pain

This patient came in with a complaint of right shoulder pain, which occurred after he had hurried through a busy airport carrying a heavy piece of luggage. His wife had referred him to Dr. Tan, as she had been successfully treated by him for her knee pain. The patient was employed in an executive level management position, a job that carried with it a considerable level of responsibility and stress. As one might guess, the shoulder injury had been the result of his struggle to keep up with the demands of his fast-paced schedule.

The patient was around 6 feet tall, and weighed 190 pounds. His pulse was slippery, and his tongue was slightly red with a thin yellow coat in the rear. He had waited for 3 months before seeking treatment, occasionally taking over-the-counter anti-inflammatory medication in hopes that the shoulder pain would resolve itself. The pain was evident upon attempting to raise his arm straight out in front of his body. It was more pronounced upon raising than lowering, and the pain was severe at about 75 degrees of frontal raising. It was not present upon abduction of the arm to the side.

For treatment, Dr. Tan inserted a needle into Stomach 41 on the right side. The insertion was deep for this point, about $3/4$ of an inch, and a good Qi sensation was generated. After about 3 minutes, he was asked to begin gently raising and lowering his shoulder while the needle was stimulated. Within a minute he was able to raise his arm up to 120 degrees before the pain bothered him. This procedure of stimulating the needle for a minute or so while the patient moved his shoulder was repeated three more times during the course of his first acupuncture treatment, which lasted about 45 minutes. The only point needled was ST41. At the conclusion of the treatment, the range of motion in his shoulder had been restored to normal and he could detect only a slight aching in the joint.

He was treated again 3 days later, at which time he described only a partial recurrence of the symptom. He was able to raise his shoulder to 120 degrees without pain, above which some pain began to occur. At the conclusion of treatment number two, his range of motion was back to normal, and this time he described the residual aching as barely perceptible. He was treated in this very simple fashion twice a week for a total of 4 weeks, when it was determined that no further treatment was needed. No recurrence of his shoulder pain has been reported since.

Summary

As a one-needle treatment, this one yielded impressive results. This case illustrates that correct point selection is more vital than the number of needles. The is what the Chinese concept "more is not necessarily better" is referring to regarding in acupuncture strategy.

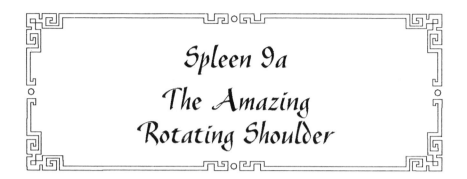

Spleen 9a
The Amazing
Rotating Shoulder

This patient had injured her left shoulder in a fall she suffered at work. She complained of severe pain and stiffness in the shoulder joint and surrounding muscles, to the degree that she was unable to sleep on her left side.

It was too painful for her to raise her arm in abduction beyond 30 percent. Rotation of the shoulder in either direction was difficult. Light palpation of the Tai Yin, Yang Ming, and Shao Yang regions of her shoulder all elicited painful responses.

The Tai Yang area was also sentitive, but to a lesser degree. Initially, Stomach 38 on the left side was palpated, found to be sensitive, and needled. A minor response was obtained—within 2 minutes the patient was able to achieve an additional 5 degrees of abduction, although there was not a noticeable improvement in rotation. Palpation of the Spleen ah shi zone on the right leg detected a reactive point approximately 1 cun below Spleen 9. Upon needling this point, a good sensation was obtained at an insertion depth of about .7 cun. At this time, both points were stimulated simultaneously while the patient again moved her shoulder. She was immediately able to abduct an additional

61

10–15 degrees. Upon the second round of point stimulus, her ability to rotate the shoulder improved markedly. During this treatment no local points were used, and after approximately 45 minutes, she was able to achieve 60 degrees of abduction, and reported a reduction of at least 70 percent in her pain symptom.

She was treated again 2 days later, at which time she reported that about 30 percent of her pain had recurred, and her shoulder abduction was at about 45 degrees. The same treatment was administered, with the Spleen 9a ah shi and ST38 being the chief points in the prescription. By the conclusion of the second treatment, her shoulder abduction had increased to approximately 90 degrees, and she rated her pain as having been reduced by 80 percent.

The third treatment was given 4 days later, and again there had been some recurrence of her pain symptom, about 20 percent. Her abduction had subsided to around 70 degrees. Overall, treatments were given at 2 day intervals, with an improvement in abduction of at least 40 degrees, and a reduction in pain of at least 60 percent. The third treatment was given 6 days after her initial visit—the points used were essentially the same. After this treatment, the patient could achieve approximately 100 degrees of abduction, and rated her pain level as being 90 percent improved. Unfortunately, at this time the patient ceased to receive acupuncture treatment for reasons that were never made clear. This eventually resulted in the need for arthroscopic surgery, from which she has yet to notice improvement comparable to that achieved from her three acupuncture treatments. Our last follow-up contact with this patient was about 7 months time following her surgery, approximately 1 year from the time of he three acupuncture treatments.

Summary

It is of interest to note that this patient had received acupuncture for her shoulder problem prior to being treated in this method, involving the use of mostly local points with electrical stimulation. In this case, one such treatment had apparently caused an aggravation of her condition, which subsided after 1 week, leaving the original degree of pain and stiffness intact. In general, any aggravation of a symptom caused by a distal point treatment will persist for a much shorter duration, usually 24–48 hours. In addition, it is typical for the patient to report an overall and sometimes dramatic improvement following the aggravation. Therefore, we have learned to look optimistically at any aggravation attributed to one of our distal point strategies.

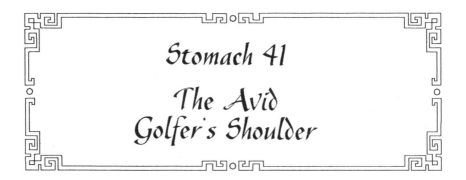

Stomach 41

The Avid Golfer's Shoulder

Golf was this fifty-five-year-old patient's passion in life. It is uncertain as to exactly how much his golf game contributed to his shoulder problem, but it definitely did not make it better. When staying away from the golf course for several weeks did not yield positive results, he decided to give acupuncture a try.

He described the pain as being in the left shoulder, deep in the joint. Upon palpation no significantly sensitive points could be detected. He experienced no problem with abduction or adduction of his arm. However, when asked to raise his straightened arm directly in front of his body, he experienced a sharp pain at about 90 degrees that radiated towards his hand. Frontal raising is considered to involve the Yang Ming channel, so the diagnosis was one of Yang Ming channel blockage. It is important to note that whenever a patient reports chest, arm, neck, or shoulder pain, especially on the left side, care should be taken to determine whether or not the heart is involved. In this case, the patient's heart was not a contributing factor.

For treatment, Stomach 41 on the left side was the main point, with Gall Bladder 40 added for assistance. On the right side

Spleen 5 was added for balance. These were the only points used in the treatment. He noticed only a slight improvement after the first treatment, but felt a significant response after treatment number two. He was able to raise his arm approximately 120 degrees before he began to feel discomfort. He was cautioned to "take it easy" and was treated with these same three points about three times a week. At treatment seven he reported feeling 90 percent better. He was able to raise his arm 180 degrees with only a slight to moderate pain.

Still, he was advised to refrain from overdoing it, and he was given some gentle stretching exercises to do. At this point, he left to spend a week in Phoenix, where the combination of his continued relief and the presence of several beautiful golf courses proved too strong a temptation for him. He succumbed to an eighteen-hole round several days in a row, causing the shoulder to be reaggravated.

Upon returning to San Diego he confessed his lapse, and treatment was commenced once again, using the same three points. This time he took the advise he was given more seriously. After another fifteen treatments in 3 weeks' time, he felt no pain or restriction of movement in his shoulder. He was advised to resume playing golf, only a few holes at first. Gradually, he was able to increase his golf game to eighteen holes without pain. After 2 years, he has not experienced any recurrence.

Summary

This case illustrates yet another good example of the need to avoid aggravating a problem during the course of treatment.

When patients feels better, it is only natural for them to think that they are in fact, completely healed; so it is up to us as the care-givers to insist upon their compliance with our instructions. In this case, the aggravation that the patient caused probably doubled the number of treatments he needed to recover adequately.

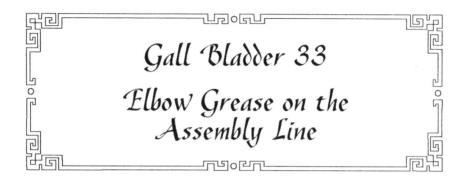

Gall Bladder 33

Elbow Grease on the Assembly Line

A fifty-five-year-old woman had a job in a factory working on an assembly line. The repetitive arm motion she employed on the line irritated her right elbow, causing soreness and swelling along the Yang Ming and Shao Yang channels. It was especially tender in the depression between the lateral epicondyle of the humerus and the olecranon, where there was also visible swelling. Palpation of the area around her left knee found Gall Bladder 33 and an ah shi point closer to the fibula were very sensitive.

These two points were needled with 30 gauge needles, obtaining a good Qi sensation. She was asked to move her elbow around during the first 10 minutes of the treatment, after which Ling Ku was needled on the right, and she was allowed to rest. (For more on the point Ling Ku, see *Twelve and Twelve in Acupuncture*, pp. 14, 15 & 48.) While the needles were in place, she could not produce the elbow pain symptom when moving her arm around. After the treatment, when the needles were out , she felt as if about 50 percent of the pain was gone. It was suggested to her that she wrap the elbow, take 3 days off of work, and receive daily treatment for those 3 days. She did this, and at the end of the 3 day period she felt no pain or stiffness in her elbow. The swelling was also reduced, there being no discernible difference between the shape and appearance of her right elbow when compared to her left. However, once she returned to work it wasn't long before the elbow became reaggravated. As a result, she needed to come for treatment twice a week for 4 weeks, before her condition began to stabilize while she continued to work. She was treated once a week for an additional 4 weeks, at which time her elbow was feeling well enough to discontinue regular treatment. She receives occasional treatment from time to time when the elbow becomes reaggravated again, usually due to working overtime on the assembly line.

Summary

In this case, as in many others, it isn't the acupuncture method or the patient's body failing to respond to treatment that prolongs the recovery, but what the patient does between treatments. Unfortunately for this person, it wasn't anything particularly fun that was causing the aggravation—it was her job.

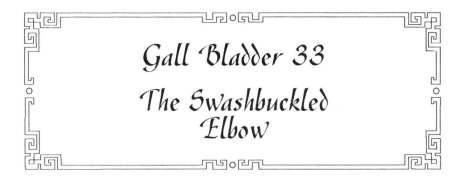

Gall Bladder 33

The Swashbuckled Elbow

A thirty-eight-year-old man came in for treatment of a tendonitis condition in his right elbow. He was a computer programmer by trade, but his interest in medieval armor is what lead to his problem. In addition to crafting replicas of medieval weaponry, he also enjoyed using it in mock sparring competitions held by a group of "Medievalists" that he belonged to. It was while practicing a move with a heavy sword, a technique taught to him by one of his comrades-in-arms, that he injured the elbow. (He later found out that this same fellow was also plagued by elbow problems.) At work, he found that prolonged use of a computer keyboard would aggravate the injury, which seemed to be keeping it from healing.

Initially, he was treated by an M.D., who administered a few cortisone shots and prescribed physical therapy along with NSAID's (non-steroidal anti-inflammatory drugs). The problem subsided for a while, but then began to slowly return. Six months after his first course of treatment, the injury had regressed to its original level of pain, swelling, and stiffness. Another course of therapy and more NSAID's were prescribed, but this time he declined to accept any further cortisone shots. Once again, some moderate relief was generated, only to disappear a few weeks after the treatment was finished. In about 4 to 6 weeks the swelling and stiffness were back to where they were they right after his injury. In addition, the NSAID's irritated his stomach. This cycle of treatment and recurrence was to be repeated two more times before he decided to come in for acupuncture treatment. The drugs and physical therapy he had received were paid for by his medical insurance, while acupuncture was not. Therefore his insurance coverage had essentially discouraged him from seeking acupuncture treatment for almost 2 years, an unfortunate situation, but one that is encountered all too frequently in this profession.

Upon examination, the patient's elbow showed visible swelling in the area of the lateral epicondyle of the humerus; i.e., along the Yang Ming and Shao Yang channels of the arm. It was very sensitive to palpation at a point just lateral to Large Intestine 11, as well as a bit proximal and distal to this point along the same channel. Flexion and extension caused pain in the swollen area especially in extension with the wrist in full extension.

The first treatment administered needling Ling Ku on the right, and three other points found in the local area of pain. (See *Twelve and Twelve* for information regarding Ling Ku and elbow treatment.) These points were all connected together with an electrical-stimulating device and set at a 2 cps. regular frequency. He reported feeling some improvement at the time of his second treatment, so the same procedure was followed. But, at the time of his third treatment he reported that the pain had reasserted itself without much improvement.

Usually, a symptom aggravation is taken as a good sign, but if it does not clear up on its own within 48 hours or so, that is another matter. In such a case it is necessary to alter the treatment strategy in an effort to lessen or eliminate the aggravation. So for treatment number three, the area around his left knee was palpated, and found to be very sensitive at the point Gall Bladder 33 and two ah shi points between the Stomach and Gall Bladder channels. These three points were needled on the left with Ling Ku on the right. A good response was obtained after about 1 minute, at which time the patient could flex and extend his elbow and wrist without pain in the elbow. The needles were left in place and stimulated at about 10 minute intervals for the duration of the treatment, which lasted about 1 hour. Each time the needles were twirled he was told to flex and extend the elbow, a technique that is intended to enhance the Qi circulating effect of the treatment in progress.

At the time of his next appointment, 5 days later, he was happily report that he was almost pain-free for 3 days. He then returned to work and aggravated it to some degree by keyboarding. Still, it was much improved, with the swelling noticeably decreased. From this point on he was treated with the same basic approach of combining Ling Ku on the right with GB33 and adjacent ah shi on the left. In addition, Spleen 9 was added on the right along with Lung 5 on the left to provide further Yin/Yang balance.

He received twenty-two additional treatments, tapering down from twice weekly in frequency to once a week, then once every 2 weeks as he continued to progress. At that point he estimated his overall improvement at better than 90 percent and had begun to carefully exercise and work with the sword again. This time he did so without the benefit of his comrade-in-arms' guidance, as the other fellow was still out of action from his elbow problems.

Summary

The first approach employed in the treatment of this case involving direct local treatment along with distal points, produced a strong aggravation of the patient's symptoms. In many cases, this can be viewed as a good sign, especially in conjunction with our mostly distal approach. Most aggravations of this sort clear themselves within 24 to 48 hours, leaving the patient feeling considerably better. As such, an aggravation constitutes something of a breakthrough in a course of treatments. But when an aggravation does not subside or is not followed by a clear sign of improvement, the treatment strategy must be changed. It was found that a distal-only strategy was the way to go in this situation. Although he required quite a few treatments to reach a state of near-total recovery, this patient did not mind; he had been through the gamut of other treatments beforehand, and knew that his was a tough case. If not for the restrictive nature of his healthcare coverage, he might have sought acupuncture treatment a lot sooner than he did, and saved himself a lot of time and suffering. As it was, he discontinued treatment before he was 100 percent recovered due to financial considerations.

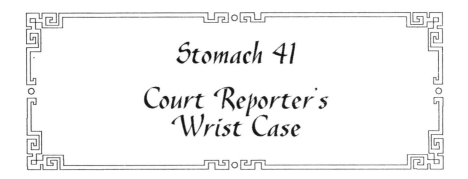

Stomach 41

Court Reporter's Wrist Case

Female, Age 32

This patient is by profession a court reporter, a job requiring a high degree of digital or manual dexterity. As with similar occupations, there is a high risk of developing overuse conditions such as carpal tunnel syndrome, which was this woman's reason for seeking acupuncture treatment from Dr. Tan. The condition was most severe in her left hand and had undergone surgery to correct it 2 years previously.

Since that time, the condition had recurred and had also developed in her right hand. No doubt this was due to the fact that she was still engaged in the same activities required at her job. In addition, she had also begun to do a lot of keyboard work at home on her computer, putting even more strain on her wrists.

For treatment, Dr. Tan chose Stomach 41 as the primary point, with Liver 3 to assist it. The points were needled bilaterally, since her condition was presenting itself that way. She was advised to slow down her pace a bit, to give her wrists a chance to rest in the evenings by cutting out all non-essential keyboard work. In all, her treatment for this condition consisted of a total of four needles per session.

Initially, she was treated three times a week for the first 3 weeks. At this time, she reported experiencing a sustained improvement in her condition that was estimated at around 70 percent. Treatment frequency was reduced to twice a week for the next 8 weeks, during which time she was still performing her full duties as a court reporter. Even though she was working, she continued to improve. At the end of 11 weeks of treatment she estimated her improvement as 90 percent. Due to her occupation, the condition continually threatens to creep back, so this patient receives two to four treatments per month to maintain her progress; she will in all probability require this for the duration of her court reporting career.

Summary

After a total of twenty-five treatments in 11 weeks' time this patient experienced a 90 percent improvement. Progress would undoubtedly have been faster if she had been able to refrain from doing activities that clearly aggravated her condition. However, in this case that would have meant staying home from work, and she simply could not afford to do so.

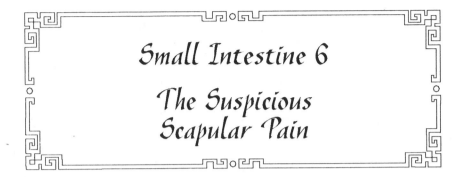

Small Intestine 6

The Suspicious
Scapular Pain

Female, Age 45

A woman complaining of neck, shoulder, and arm pain came to the school clinic at the American Institute of Oriental Medicine. At the time, Steve was on duty as clinic supervisor. The intern assigned to treat this woman was alarmed by the case, and understandably so. The patient's symptoms were presenting on the left side, and she had a history of angina, taking a prescribed sublingual nitroglycerin tablet as needed. That week, she had such acute pain she was taken to the emergency room , where a total of three EKG's were performed. All of them failed to detect any abnormality. Upon questioning her further it became apparent that her angina pains were suspected to be due to a vascular spasm phenomena, rather than to a narrowed coronary arterial lumen. Her blood pressure was measured at 130/90. For her pain, the emergency room doctor had prescribed Vicodin, a powerful pain medication that actually afforded little or no relief from her suffering.

Careful examination of the patient revealed that the area of neck pain and stiffness was in both the Shao Yang and Tai Yang

75

zones on the left side and was primarily rotational in nature. There was no actual pain along the course of the carotid artery, however. The pain traveled further down the course of the left Tai Yang line to the lower border of the scapula. It was also discovered that she was not actually suffering from pain along the left arm, but rather a sort of vague tingling sensation which she seemed to experience intermittently. Furthermore, she reported that none of her symptoms were aggravated by exercise at her health club. In light of these findings, it seemed as if her pain was more of a channel, or Qi stagnation type, than due to a heart organ dysfunction. Therefore, Steve determined that it was safe to treat her with acupuncture.

For treatment, the points Heart 4 and Gall Bladder 39 on the right, with San Jiao 5 and Spleen 6 on the left were suggested. (For more information concerning our use of these points, please see our first book, *Twelve and Twelve in Acupuncture*.) Upon stimulus of these points, her rotational neck pain diminished immediately. However, after checking with her a few minutes later, she reported that the pain in the area of her scapula was still present. Steve suggested that SJ5 on the left be changed to Small Intestine 6, with the needle pointing in the direction of the channel flow. Upon obtaining a Qi sensation from this point, the patient felt an immediate relief from the pain in her scapula area. In addition to the four needles used, the intern treating this patient also administered about 5 to 10 minutes of Tui Na (Chinese massage) to the Tai Yang area of her upper back while the needles were in place. This helped to further reduce the Qi stagnation in the area, and the patient left the clinic her condition greatly improved.

Summary

Acupuncture is one of the safest healing modalities that can be employed, but of course, it is still necessary to determine to your complete satisfaction that the patient is stable enough to receive treatment. This is especially true if there is no emergency equipment and/or appropriately trained personnel on hand to deal with an emergency such as cardiac arrest. This patient continued to come in for weekly treatment after her first visit, and after several weeks reported that her overall condition, including the angina, was much better.

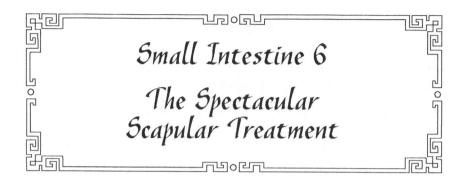

Small Intestine 6
The Spectacular Scapular Treatment

Female, Age 56

A 56-year-old woman employed in a manufacturing job came in complaining of pain in her right upper back, radiating down her right arm to her wrist. Upon examination, it was found that she was sensitive to palpation of the point Small Intestine 11 and the Tai Yang area of her right upper back, especially along the medial border of her right scapula. The radiating pain was found to involve the Small Intestine channel on the upper arm, switching to the San Jiao channel on the lower arm. Posterior extension of her arm aggravated the pain.

For treatment, Dr. Tan chose Small Intestine 6 as the primary point, needling it on the same (right) side as the pain. Spleen 6 was also needled on the right side. On the left side, the points Heart 4 and Gall Bladder 39 provided an energetic balance. She had never experienced acupuncture before and was a little nervous, as well as curious about the fact that there were no needles placed in the vicinity of her actual aches and pains. After reassuring her, Dr. Tan then connected SI6 to SP6 with an electrical-stimulator, set to a low frequency (2 cps.). He did the same with

HT4 and GB39. The patient was then left to relax for about 40 minutes.

At the conclusion of the treatment, the patient reported being pain-free. She returned for her next appointment 3 days later, stating that after her first treatment she had remained completely pain-free for a period of around 4 hours, after which some of the symptoms began to slowly return. Until the second treatment the pain had not returned to its original level, being only about half as intense as it originally was. The same treatment was performed again. She was also pain-free at the conclusion of this treatment.

Upon returning for treatment number three, 4 days later, she told us that the total relief had lasted for an entire day before any of the pain began to return. At this time only about 20 percent of the original level of pain remained, but the patient was able to detect a soreness in the right shoulder joint which she hadn't noticed before. To address this, Stomach 41 on the right side was added to the treatment. This relieved the pain in her shoulder joint. She reported feeling fine after her treatment and did not return for another appointment until the following week.

Her condition at that time had been aggravated due to her job activities. The pain was still less than 50 percent than before she received acupuncture treatment. She was treated with the original four needle combination, as well as with the electrical-stimulator. This patient received two more treatments, for a total of six. One year after the completion of her course of treatment, her shoulder was still pain-free.

Summary

In this case, the point SI6 was the principle point used to address the patient's scapular pain. When she also noticed pain in the shoulder joint itself, ST41 was added. We have found that both of these points tend to be most effective distally when needled on the same side as the pain, which amounts to something of a divergence from our standard of contralateral needling. The electrical stimulator in this case served to make a stronger energetic connection between the points without having to generate too strong a Qi sensation.

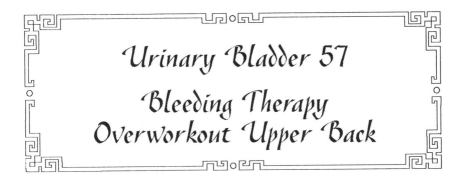

Urinary Bladder 57
Bleeding Therapy
Overworkout Upper Back

Female, Age 24

After a strenuous workout at her health club, this twenty-four-year-old woman experienced a sharp pain in her upper back. When the pain did not diminish after 2 days, she came in to be treated.

Upon examination, the pain was found to be centered at the level of the seventh and eigth thoracic vertebrae, both sides of the spine being more or less equally sensitive to palpation. Any movement in this area aggravated the pain, often causing it to radiate to the ribs. Palpation of the Urinary Bladder line on her lower legs found sensitive spots in the UB57 area on both legs. On the left leg a large number of purplish capillaries were noted.

Since the pain in her upper back was bilateral, a bilateral treatment was indicated. Instead of needling, both of these points were bled. On the left, it was easy to induce a good bleeding response when the capillaries were punctured with a lancet. On the right, however, the puncture alone released very little blood, so a cup was applied to draw out more. She was able to feel the sharpness and tension in her upper back decrease almost instantly when this was done. The pain was almost totally gone when she left the office.

Her second treatment was 3 days later, at which time she reported that the residual pain was only about a third of what it originally was. Upon inspection, there was still some visible capillary distention in the UB57 region, so once again the bleeding technique was applied. She was also told to use a heating pad on the area when she was at home in the evenings. She called the day before her third appointment to cancel, as all of the pain was gone and had not returned.

Summary

Bleeding alone was sufficient in this case to treat the patient's pain and stagnation symptoms. Just as UB40 is known for its relationship to the lower back region, so we have found UB57 to relate to the upper back. In a somewhat tougher case, this bleeding technique might have been used as an opener for an acupuncture treatment involving distal and/or local points. Of course, the proper precautions should always be taken whenever a risk of exposure to a patient's blood is involved. Rubber gloves are essential, but they provide no protection against an accidental needle stick. There is no substitute for mindfulness when performing acupuncture or bleeding therapy!

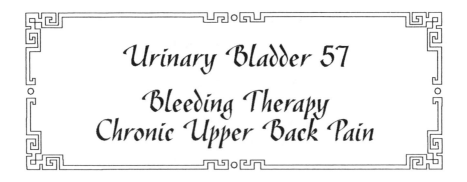

Urinary Bladder 57
Bleeding Therapy
Chronic Upper Back Pain

A seventy-five-year-old woman with a history of high blood pressure came in for treatment of upper back pain that had been bothering her for several weeks. Upon examination, it was noted that the pain seemed to be centered around the sixth and seventh thoracic area. It was presented on both sides of the spine, but was worse on the left.

For the first treatment, Chung Tze and Chung Hsien were used on the right side, along with Ling Ku. (See *Twelve and Twelve in Acupuncture* for more information on this dynamic point combination.) Surprisingly, there was little or no improvement from this normally very effective point prescription. Upon her return two days later, the areas along her Urinary Bladder channel on the lower legs were palpated and inspected; and a number of bluish black capillaries was detected in the UB57 area of her left leg. The patient's blood pressure visit was 170/100. With the patient lying in a prone position, the bluish capillaries in the UB57 area were pricked for bleeding. She reported a sensation of immediate pain relief, estimating it as an almost 50 percent improvement. Following the bleeding, she was asked to turn over, and the previous treatment (Chung Tze-Hsien and Ling

Ku) was once again administered. This time good results were obtained. She left the office that day feeling much better.

For the course of her treatment, she came in twice a week. For the next 4 weeks, the points being used were essentially the same. The bleeding technique was repeated every three to four treatments, or whenever significantly pronounced veins showed up in the UB57 area. After eleven treatments the pain was completely gone and did not recur.

Summary

On occasion, one of our favorite point prescriptions will fail to do its characteristically good job, even though it seems to be the point combination indicated. In such cases, it is always helpful to examine the appropriate areas of the body where capillary stagnation may be related to the patient's problem, and to bleed the capillaries if they stand out. This, of course is not our original finding as the Nei Ching itself notes that "Chronic blockages can be cleared by bleeding." We have simply expanded our knowledge of how to apply this theory with different distal point methods.

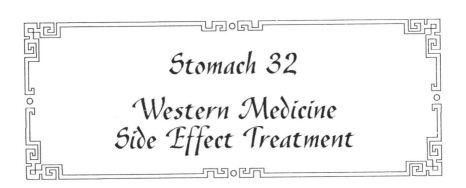

Stomach 32

Western Medicine
Side Effect Treatment

A thirty-year-old female, diagnosed as being hypothyroid, came in for treatment complaining of heartburn and palpitations, a common side effect of the thyroid medication she was taking. To counteract the side effect, her M.D. had prescribed another drug, Tagamet. The symptoms were usually worse just before her menstruation. Due to her extreme fear of needles, only two needles were used for the first treatment—Stomach 36 and Spleen 9. She experienced no pain after her first treatment for 3 days. (Very sensitive and/or nervous patients often experience unusually strong responses to acupuncture treatment.) She still experienced some heartburn sensations as well as some palpitations afterwards.

For her second treatment, Stomach 32 was needled alone on the left side, remaining in place alone for 2 minutes, at which time she reported feeling no further palpitations. Then points SP9 and San Jiao 5 on the right, along with Stomach 36 and Percardium 6 on the left were added. They were left in place for another 15 to 20 minutes, at which time she experienced no symptoms at all. There was no recurrence.

Summary

This was a two treatment case in which severe drug side effects were successfully treated with acupuncture. In fact, further treatment probably could have helped her thyroid condition as well.

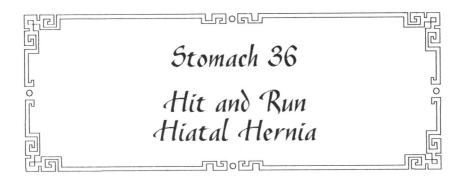

Stomach 36

Hit and Run
Hiatal Hernia

Female, Age 56

Never suspecting that she had a hernia, this patient's first acquaintance with it was a memorable one. Instead of the more typical pattern of gradually worsening symptoms, this one hit her like a truck! After climbing up three flights of stairs, she experienced severe difficulty in breathing and subsequently fainted. Other symptoms which presented themselves at this time were profuse sweating and pallor. It would therefore come as no surprise to find that the emergency room staff treated her as a heart attack case when she first arrived. However, repeated EKG and blood tests found no sign of heart trouble. Further testing detected the hiatal hernia, and it was determined to be the cause of her fainting. It seems that the combination of discomfort from the hernia, along with its restriction of her normal deep breathing capacity, caused her to experience a kind of shock. Prior to this rather dramatic event, she had only noticed an occasional feeling of discomfort before or after eating, but paid little attention to it.

The severity of her symptoms increased after this dramatic event, but did not again culminate with fainting. They were severe enough for her to consult with us, however, having been referred by her chiropractor, who was also one of our patients. Upon examination, the patient's pulse was found to be shi (excess in the guan, or middle) position on the right, with Kidney deficiency showing itself on the left. Indeed, the patient did report some chronic low back pain as well, which is a typical sign of Kidney deficiency. Her tongue was swollen with toothmarks.

For treatment, Stomach 36 was needled on the left side, with Spleen 9 on the right. Pericardium 6 was needled on the left arm and San Jiao 5 on the right. Thus, we were employing the "Tai Qi" strategy of polarizing the limbs by using only Yin or Yang points on opposing arms and legs. This increases Qi circulation throughout the body, an important factor in the treatment of chronic con-ditions. Within minutes, the discomfort had disappeared. She did experience a degree of recurrence between treatments, but overall the severity steadily decreased. After the fourteenth treatment she had no further symptoms. Six more treatments were administered, after which the patient reported no recurrence in a year's time.

Summary

In Traditional Chinese medical theory, all manner of lumps, protrusions, and swellings can be treated. In the case of hernia, we cannot say exactly what takes place during a successful series of treatments. But, as in this case, the result was a good one. We have also successfully used distal point theory to treat calcaneal spurs. In two cases, we were fortunate enough to obtain before and after x-rays that confirmed the patient's improvement. (Please see *Twelve and Twelve in Acupuncture* for more information on the treatment of heel spurs.)

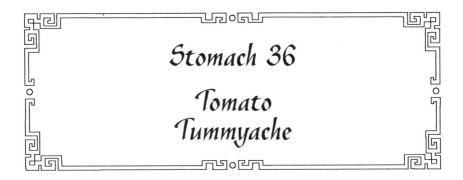

Stomach 36

Tomato Tummyache

A sixty-eight-year-old woman came to Dr. Tan with a 7 year history of hiatal hernia pain. A likable, easygoing woman, she had been referred to the doctor by her friend, a church organist. She also suffered from headaches and eye problems. She reported the stomach pain as being aggravated just prior to and following a meal. A bloating sensation would often accompany the post-meal pain. Her pulse was excess in the guan (middle) position, and her tongue exhibited dryness with a slight coat in the center.

For treatment, Stomach 36 was selected as the chief point. It was needled on the left along with Spleen 10. On the left arm, San Jiao 5 was chosen. On the right leg, ST34 and SP9 were the points used. Percardium 6 was needled on the right arm. A good Qi sensation was obtained on all the needles. The pain began to subside within 5 minutes and was completely gone before the end of her first treatment. After five treatments, the pain ceased to recur unless the patient ate spaghetti or some other food with tomato sauce. Naturally, Dr. Tan advised her to avoid all such foods. The patient found that as long as she followed this advice, her stomach pain did not return.

Summary

Two noteworthy items are illustrated in this case. First, Dr. Tan did not follow his somewhat characteristic "Tai Qi" strategy—the principle of "polarizing" the limbs (i.e., needling only yin points on one leg and yang points on the other), a strategy he frequently employs when treating chronic conditions. Instead, he created a mini-Tai Qi balance on each leg itself, using SP9 to balance ST34 and SP10 to balance ST36. However, on the arms we can see the now familiar arrangement of P6 across from SJ5.

Second, although not necessarily curing the patient's hiatal hernia, this treatment approach was able to greatly decrease the actual symptoms. After the course of treatment, patient had problems only when she ate offending foods . . . such as tomato sauce.

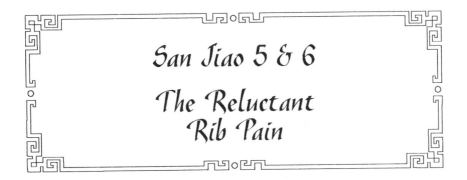

San Jiao 5 & 6

The Reluctant Rib Pain

Female, Age 42

This is a case in which the patient suffered with her complaint for some time, before successfully coping with her fear of needles and trying acupuncture for her costal pain. Unfortunately, it seems that she did not also harbor a phobia towards scalpels; during the time preceding her acupuncture treatment, she submitted to surgery on no fewer than seven occasions. Although the surgeries she had undergone were for problems other than rib pain, another operation was scheduled to address that condition. Since her mother was a patient of Dr. Tan's and had experienced excellent results from his acupuncture treatment for a variety of problems, she decided it was time, at last, to give it a try.

The patient complained of pain that was severe at times, in her right costal region just below the breast, and also in the upper chest. She had been experiencing this pain for the last year-and-a-half, but had avoided seeing the acupuncturist because of her needle phobia. Her pulse was superficial and wiry, her tongue dusky.

For treatment, San Jiao 5 and 6 were selected for treatment on the right side, and on the left Gall Bladder 34 was the only point used. In spite of her anxiety, she was able to tolerate a fairly substantial Qi sensation on this, her first treatment. The result was astonishing to her, but not too surprising to the doctor. About 1 minute after the needles' insertion, she began to notice a reduction in her pain, which at the time of her treatment, she had estimated as being towards the severe end of its spectrum.

The pain continued to subside, and by the end of her first treatment about 45 minutes later, she reported feeling pain-free for the first time in years. She could not contain herself and burst into tears right there on the treatment table. Of course, Dr. Tan was happy too, but his response, feigning sternness, was to ask her why she hadn't come to see him sooner.

In all, the patient received three more treatments, for a total of four, administered over a 3 week period. To date, she reports no recurrence.

Summary

After only four treatments, this patient was relieved of a pain that had bothered her for over 1 year, and for which an exploratory surgery had already been scheduled. Interestingly, even though she expressed some fear of the acupuncture needles, she was able to tolerate a fairly strong Qi sensation with no problem...a major factor in the quick resolution of this case. She continues to receive periodic treatment for general wellness and other concerns, having realized through her experience that acupuncture needles are actually less scary than scalpels!

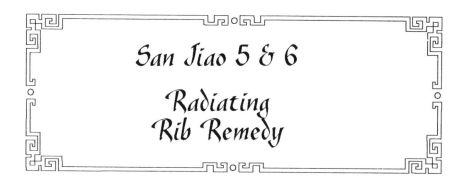

San Jiao 5 & 6

Radiating
Rib Remedy

Female, Age 55

A 55-year-old woman came to see Dr. Tan complaining of pain in the right chest and costal region. Medical tests conducted to discover the source of the pain had all proven negative. The patient was significantly overweight. She was especially bothered by this pain due to the fact that it interfered with her sleep, making her feel tired during the day. The pain had been bothering her for at least 6 months. At times the pain would radiate around to her mid-back area. Right side costal pain which radiates to the back or scapular region is a common symptom of Gall Bladder problems; however, the findings from her lab tests were negative. Upon palpation of the area on her back, it was determined that the Gall Bladder Shu point was not the area most sensitive, and that no specific Shu point was the center of the radiating pain. Rather, the sensitivity was between Shu points, although definitely on the Urinary Bladder channel. Her pulse was wiry and a little tight.

For treatment, San Jiao 5 and 6 were needled on the right side, along with an ah shi point in the area of SJ9. The only point needled on the left side was Urinary Bladder 58. Since the pain radiated towards the Urinary Bladder channel in general, with no specific Shu point being particularly involved, UB58, the Luo point, was chosen. After needling the above mentioned four points and obtaining a significant, but moderate Qi sensation at each point, the UB channel area was again palpated. At a bit more than 1 minute's time into the treatment, the sensitivity in this area was gone.

These four points provided the core treatment strategy in this case. In all, she received two such treatments a week for a 6 week period. At the time of the final treatment, she reported having experienced no recurrence of her pain for over 2 weeks.

Summary

After failing to diagnose the source of this patient's pain with standard medical tests (x-rays, blood work, etc.), her problem was still fairly easy to treat with acupuncture. By viewing it as a Qi stagnation phenomena and treating it according to channel theory, a 6-month-old problem was cleared up in 6 weeks.

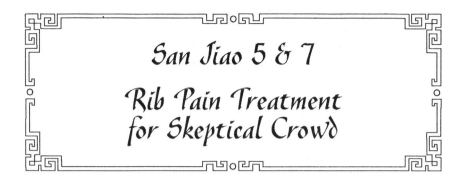

San Jiao 5 & 7
Rib Pain Treatment for Skeptical Crowd

At a recent seminar that Dr. Tan gave, part of the presentation involved actual demonstration treatments given to patients brought in by the participants themselves. On this occasion, one such demo treatment was to function as quite an eye-opener for a number of the attending practitioners.

Many of the acupuncturists had expressed doubts about the possibility of distal point treatment alone being sufficient to effectively treat a stubborn pain problem. Others were also particularly skeptical about the likelihood of distal points on the extremities being used to effectively treat trunk or abdominal pain and stagnation. Still others, attributing the effects of acupuncture to the relatively limited known actions of the endorphin mechanism, found the idea of almost instant pain relief hard to believe, probably since the scientific research that exists concerning the topic seems to indicate that endorphin release occurs more slowly (a 15 to 30 minute latency period in the case of acupuncture experiments). All of the doubters felt that local points would have to be added in order to obtain a beneficial response.

The first patient to be treated that afternoon dramatically challenged their perspectives on these issues. She was a twenty-five-year-old female who had been suffering for several weeks from right-sided rib pain, just below her breast. Conventional medical testing found no underlying pathology. She described the pain as more or less constant, on occasion radiating back towards her spine. Asked to rate her pain on a scale of one to ten, with ten being the most severe, she rated her pain level at the time of this treatment as a seven. This was to be her first acupuncture treatment.

Upon palpation of the San Jiao channel, the points SJ5 and 7 were found to be very tender and reactive on her left arm. As she sat on a couch facing the audience, these two points were needled, obtaining a moderate Qi sensation. (This was, after all, her first acupuncture treatment.) Within 5 seconds the patient was amazed to find that the pain was not present when she breathed in deeply, and within 30 seconds she reported that it seemed to have disappeared altogether.

The skeptical practitioners in the audience maintained a steady flow of questions all throughout her treatment, asking if the pain was coming back, or if it had moved to another place, etc. Finally, they were all convinced and had to admit that Dr. Tan had shown them something new and impressive. The needles were left in place for at least 20 more minutes, and when they were removed the pain did not return. Everyone, including the patient, was impressed by this demonstration. It is our sincere hope that their willingness to be more open-minded concerning this subject endures to this day.

Summary

It is perhaps considered common knowledge by many practitioners that the San Jiao channel can be used to treat rib pain. We have found, however, that if the pain to be treated is unilateral, then unilateral application of the San Jiao points will prove far more effective than bilateral needling. Exactly which side to use remains the question to be answered. Usually the opposite or contralateral San Jiao points will be more sensitive to palpation; this indicates the most effective side to needle.

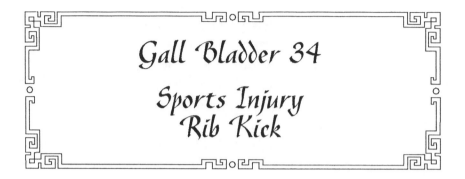

Gall Bladder 34

Sports Injury
Rib Kick

A twenty-eight-year-old man was waiting in front of the clinic one morning before opening time. He was suffering from an acute injury to his rib area and was there as a walk-in to obtain treatment for the pain. The day before he had been playing in a soccer game when he was accidentally kicked in his rib area on his right side, just below the nipple. He went to the emergency room of a nearby hospital that night. X-rays were taken, but proved negative for possible fractures. Nonetheless, he had sustained a severe bruise which was quite painful which greatly restricted his movement. He knew that acupuncture was effective for treating injuries, so he decided after a difficult night to come to the office first thing in the morning.

Upon moderately deep inhalation, he experienced a dull ache in the area of his injury. It was understandably very tender to palpation. His pulse was wiry and tight. Upon palpation of the Gall Bladder channel, Gall Bladder 34 was found to be very sensitive on the left side. GB33 was also very tender, so both points were selected and needled together on the left side. A thicker 30 gauge needle was selected for both points, in order to obtain a good strong Qi sensation. After the needles were in place, and while they were being stimulated, he was again asked to try to take a deep breath. To his amazement, he found that the dull ache was not there. The two needles were then left in place, being stimulated at about 10 minute intervals over a 90 minute period. At the end of his first treatment, he felt that about seventy percent of the pain was gone. He was given some capsules of Yunnan Baiyao, a Chinese herbal formula that is good for traumatic injuries, and sent home with instructions to return the next day. The same two needle treatment was repeated twice more on consecutive days. After three treatments there was no further discernible pain in the area. The bruise had resolved itself to a greenish color and the remainder of his injury resolved itself within a few days.

Summary

This is another relatively simple case of what we might refer to as "Sports Acupuncture" in action. In the future, acupuncture techniques like these will play an important role in the increasing use of acupuncture and acupuncturists by athletes and sports organizations.

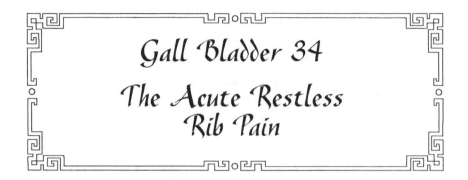

Gall Bladder 34
The Acute Restless Rib Pain

Female, Age 34

This patient presented with acute right-sided rib pain. She described the pain as radiating to her back, in the lower thoracic region. She also reported feelings of nausea and indigestion, with a slight bitter taste in her mouth. She was very irritable and restless, and her pulse was wiry and tight. Initially, she had been treated for stress and low resistance to colds and flu. Recently she had been fighting a vaginal yeast infection for 2 weeks, which had been resolved. Prior to that she was sick with flu-like symptoms for 3 days. Her condition at the time of this visit constituted a classic example of Liver and Gall Bladder Qi stagnation. Had the pain presented itself as severe with extreme sensitivity upon palpation, one might suspect gallstones as the cause. As it was, the condition appeared to be one that involved a Qi stagnation, or a less advanced state of imbalance than one resulting from stones. (Needless to say, if there is ever any doubt at all, the acupuncturist is ethically and legally obligated to refer a patient for immediate medical evaluation of such a condition.)

A total of four needles were chosen for treatment in this case. The principle point selected was Gall Bladder 34, applied contralaterally. Opposite GB34, on the right side, Liver 7 was used to provide a yin/yang balance. On the upper limb, the points selected were Pericardium 6 on the left and San Jiao 5 on the right. An electrical-stimulating device was employed to connect GB34 with P6, and LV7 with SJ5. The setting was a continuous signal set at 1 cycle per second. The patient experienced noticeable relief within the first minute of treatment, with all of the pain gone after 20 minutes' time. The patient has reported no recurrence since then.

Summary

As the results obtained from this treatment reveal, the patient's problem was Qi stagnation rather than blood stagnation or a stone. All licensed acupuncturists receive adequate training to differentiate between such conditions, but actual clinical experience is invaluable in order to make such decisions with confidence. This point combination is also very effective in the treatment of chronic rib pain.

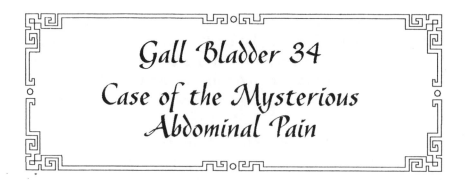

Gall Bladder 34
Case of the Mysterious
Abdominal Pain

Female, Age 25

After seeing her M.D. and receiving tests in an unsuccessful attempt to discover the cause of her lower abdominal pain, this patient of came in for treatment. She had been a patient of Dr. Tan's previously, having been successfully treated for a variety of health problems.

The pain was located in the right lower abdominal area, and the points Spleen 14, Liver 13, and Gall Bladder 26 were all noticeably more sensitive to palpation on the right side. The abdominal pain had been present for approximately 3 weeks, the patient being unable to pinpoint the exact time that it first occurred. She was also unable to associate any incident or event leading to its onset. She reported the pain was aggravated by running, and that at times it seemed to radiate upwards towards her ribs. The pain was making her quite irritable, which resulted in considerable stress in her professional and personal life. Her pulse was wiry, and her tongue was red around the edges. All of these signs pointed to a classic case of Liver and Gall Bladder Qi stagnation.

For treatment, the principle point selected was Gall Bladder 34 on the right side.

Dr. Tan has found this point effective contralaterally in treating rib pain, while it is more effective on the same side in the treatment of pain in the lower abdomen. In both instances, this point is indicated whenever Liver and Gall Bladder Qi stagnation is suspected as a cause or major contributing factor. On her left leg, Liver 5 was the only point needled. The other two needles employed in this treatment were Pericardium 6 and San Jiao 5, on the right and left sides respectively. The pain disappeared after about 5 minutes into the treatment. The needles were left in place for approximately 45 minutes. (This is a fairly average length of time for one of Dr. Tan's treatments.) She was given the Chinese patent herbal formula "Shu Kan Wan" (Hepato-Tonic Pills), to take three times daily. At the time of her next visit 3 days later, she reported that although the pain had not returned, she could still detect a slight "twitching" sensation in the area at times. The same treatment was repeated with the same positive results being obtained. No further treatment was given.

Summary

In all, the course of treatment for this case consisted of four acupuncture treatments in 10 days' time. She reported no recurrence of this symptom after 6 months.

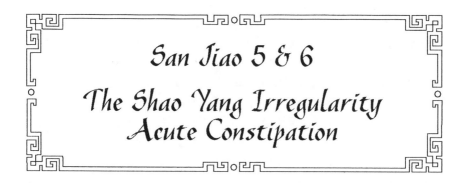

San Jiao 5 & 6
The Shao Yang Irregularity
Acute Constipation

Female, Age 35

This is an interesting but brief case study involving an episode of acute constipation. The patient, an otherwise fit and active woman, presented with symptoms of costal distention on the right side and constipation. She had been without a bowel movement for approximately 48 hours. She felt "stuck" in her abdomen—the middle jiao area. She reported difficulty sleeping, irritability, and was experiencing skin breakout on her face and neck. Her pulse was full, wiry, and slightly fast. Her tongue was reddish with some coating in the central rear area. In Zhang/Fu terms, she was presenting as a case of Liver and Gall Bladder Qi stagnation with some heat signs as well.

For treatment, the points San Jiao 5 and 6 were selected on the left side. SJ6 is well known for its effect on the colon, but we find its effect in this regard greatly enhanced by the addition of SJ5, right next to it. On the right arm these were balanced with Pericardium 6. P6 was a good choice here not only because of its functions for calming spirit, harmonizing the center, and clearing heat, but also because Jue Yin balances Shao Yang so well.

The names of SJ5 and P6—Waiguan and Neiguan (Outer and Inner Gates, respectively)—also reveal the special balance that can be attained between these two points. For the lower limbs, Stomach 37 was selected on the right side and Kidney 6 on the left. ST37, of course, is the lower He-Sea point for the large intestine, and K6 has a fairly well-known ability to "open" the intestines. By selecting the points in this fashion, a good Yin/Yang polarity was achieved in both the horizontal (left to right) and vertical (hand to foot) planes. A proper Qi sensation was obtained from all of the points, and within 1 minute or so of inserting the needle, the patient began to experience an increasing number of bowel sounds and feelings of movement. After about 30 minutes into the treatment time, the needles had to be removed a bit early, as the patient was in a hurry to visit the restroom!

Summary

In this case, the principle points, San Jiao 5 and 6, worked very quickly to move the patient's Qi stagnation. This combination also works very well when applied in the treatment of more chronic conditions of constipation.

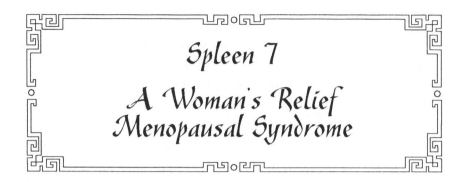

Spleen 7
A Woman's Relief
Menopausal Syndrome

A forty-eight-year-old woman who was in good health otherwise, came in with complaints about irregular menstruation. Its onset had been in the last 2 months; her menses were accompanied by painful cramps, mostly on the right side, which she had never suffered from before. At times, the pain would be severe enough to nauseate her and cause her to vomit. She did not wish to continue with the over-the-counter medications she was using because the drugs had little or no positive effect on her suffering.

Upon examination, her pulse on the left was found to be slippery and strong in the Kidney position, while being deficient and deep on the right. This disparity between Kidney pulses in such a case means that the hormonal system is seriously out of balance. For verification purposes (and to satisfy insurance company requirements), she was sent for a blood test to measure hormone levels. According to the test, she was beginning menopause.

Before treatment, a strong ah shi point was located along the Spleen channel very close to Spleen 7. SP6 and 9 were also found to be very sensitive. The ah shi was especially strong on the left side, contralateral to the pain in her right lower abdomen. These three points were needled on the left with the point Stomach 40 used on the right for balance. Within 10 minutes of needle insertion, the abdominal pain ceased. The needles were left in place for a total of approximately forty-five minutes. She was treated twice a week initially, decreasing the treatment frequency as her condition improved. She had also begun experiencing hot flashes and night sweats, both of which decreased as the treatments were repeated. After ten treatments the pains disappeared, not to recur. It was recommended that she continue to come in once a week for treatment to help prevent further complications from her menopause.

Summary

Menstruation problems are often related to the Spleen, especially if irregular or very heavy periods are occurring. Even though her condition was initially noticed via her Kidney pulses, this is still often the case. The discovery of the extra sensitivity along Spleen channel points helped to verify the fact that her Spleen was the key imbalance contributing to this situation.

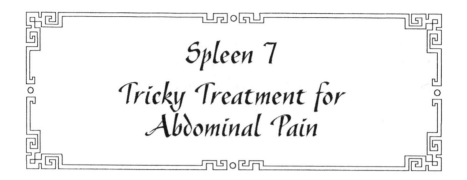

Spleen 7
Tricky Treatment for Abdominal Pain

A forty-four-year-old woman had been experiencing menopause symptoms for over a year. She had ceased menstruation in the last 6 months, and her hot flashes and emotional mood swings had been reduced to some degree by estrogen replacement. She also had been taking an oral estrogen medication for the 2 months prior to coming into the acupuncture clinic. What brought her in to try acupuncture was an excruciating pain that had occurred in her right lower abdomen 2 days earlier. The pain was so intense that it caused her to break into a cold sweat, and she was taken to a nearby hospital emergency room for help. Several tests were conducted, but as no cause could be ascertained, the doctors were unable to arrive at a diagnosis. She was given an injection which decreased the pain to a degree, and sent home with no further treatment. The following morning when she found the pain returning, she decided to come in for acupuncture.

Upon examination, her pulse was wiry, and the area of sensitivity on her abdomen appeared to be along the Spleen channel on the right side of her lower abdomen. A very sensitive ah shi point on the left leg in the vicinity of Spleen 7 was located; SP6 and SP9 were also being sensitive to palpation. On the right leg, a point near Stomach 39 was found to be sensitive as well.

For treatment, a strong Qi sensation was necessary in this case, so a 30 gauge Chinese needle was selected. The first point needled was the Spleen 7 ah shi, and a strong Qi sensation was indeed generated, causing the patient to scream! However, 1 minute later, the pain began to diminish—a phenomenon which she attributed to being "some kind of trick." Dr. Tan replied, "If it works, who cares if it's a trick?" The other two Spleen points were then needled, followed by the Stomach 39 ah shi point on the right leg. In all, only four needles were used. The needles were twirled every 5 to 10 minutes, and at the end of the treatment, about an hour later, the pain was completely gone.

The next day, she reported that the pain had returned overnight, only this time it was not as intense—reduced to only a dull ache. Her pulse was wiry and rolling, suggesting that she would soon have another menstrual period—her first in over 6 months. The treatment given this time consisted only of the SP7 ah shi on the left and the ST39 ah shi on the right. At the end of this treatment, the dull ache was completely gone. The next day, her menstruation did indeed start in the morning. Initially, there were many dark clots, followed by a more normal flow. After this short menstrual period, she felt much better overall. Returning for a follow-up treatment a week later, she was given only an herbal formula, because acupuncture was no longer necessary in this case.

Summary

Abdominal pain during menopause is a common event. Even when undiagnosable in Western medical terms, it can still be treated effectively with Chinese medicine by following channel theory. In this case the pain was quite strong, which required a strong stimulus at the acupuncture points used for treatment.

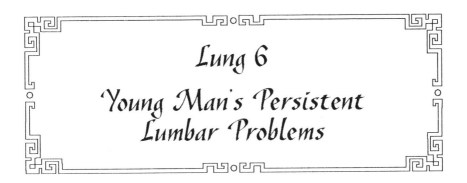

Lung 6
'Young Man's Persistent Lumbar Problems

A twenty-five-year-old male, whose chief complaint was of a persistent upper lumbar pain (duration of at least 6 months), came in for treatment. Upon examination it was found to be distributed between the first lumbar and eleventh thoracic vertebrae, more or less bilaterally. When aggravated it would radiate both upwards and downwards along the Urinary Bladder channel. He was unable to recall exactly how or when the pain had originated, but assumed that he had caused it himself from over-exertion at any one of his many athletic activities.

For treatment, the Ling Ku combination was employed for the first four sessions. (See our previous book, *Twelve and Twelve in Acupuncture* for further information on this point combination.) These treatments cleared up most of his back pain, but he still felt some stiffness upon rising in the morning as well as some aching in the area after a long day. Lying face down on the treatment table seemed to make it worse, so he was treated in one of the clinic's four reclining "Lazy-Boy" chairs. Upon palpation of his upper forearm, the Lung 6 points were found to be especially sensitive; an ah shi point between LU6 and 5 was very tender as well. These four points were needled bilaterally and were stimulated at 10 minute intervals throughout the treatment. They were needled rather deeply, at about 1 to 1.5 cun. The treatment lasted just under an hour, at which time he reported being almost pain-free. Upon returning 2 days later, his after-work soreness had been reduced dramatically, with an improvement in his early morning stiffness as well. LU6 was needled again, along with Urinary Bladder 40.

Returning for his next treatment a few days later, his symptoms were reduced to only a slight sensation of stiffness, as well as an occasional "twitching" sensation in the area. The same treatment was given. When he returned the following week, he estimated his improvement overall as at least 80 percent. Some low back pain in the fourth and fifth lumbar area had resurfaced, however. For this treatment, the left side was needled with the Ling Ku combination and Kidney 3. The right was treated with LU6 ah shi and UB40 for a leg point. On his next visit, his ninth treatment for this condition, he reported having remained pain free with only a small amount of residual stiffness upon rising in the morning. The same treatment was given again. Two additional treatments were given over the next 3 weeks to consolidate the effect. He reported no further problems with his lower back.

Summary

In all, this was an eleven-treatment case. The number of needles used per treatment varied from four to six, depending on which strategy was being employed. The strategy varied from time to time according to the way that his symptoms were presenting themselves.

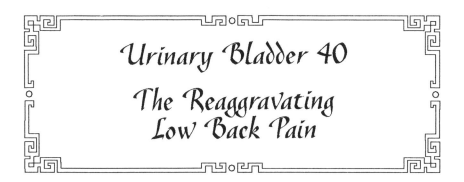

Urinary Bladder 40
The Reaggravating Low Back Pain

Female, Age 55

Having been diagnosed by an M.D. over 3 years ago as suffering from advanced arthritis in the lumbar spine, this patient began acupuncture treatment almost immediately, experiencing a great degree of relief. She had also been successfully treated during this time for neck and scapular pain.

However, one day while doing some work around the house, she aggravated the lower back problem again by pulling on a heavy piece of furniture. When she came in for treatment, the right side of her lumbar region appeared raised and swollen and was very sensitive to palpation. The area most affected was along the Urinary Bladder channel on the right side, between UB23 and UB25 (Lumbar 2–5). Upon further examination, the area around UB40 exhibited a few very dark veins, which are regarded as a sign of Qi and blood stagnation in the lower back.

Using a standard disposable bleeding lancet, the darkest of these veins was punctured. The stagnation in that particular vein was so strong that it caused the blood to spurt out almost 2 feet into the air. In all, two or three spots in the area of UB40 on both legs were pricked. Immediately after, the patient reported feeling a definite improvement in her lower back. Following the bleeding, a standard Traditional Chinese Medicine treatment was administered: UB40, UB60, and local points were needled. At the end of her treatment, she was once again pain free.

Summary

Even patients who have been successfully treated for a condition and have remained stable for a long time can experience a recurrence of their symptoms due to an accident or some other type of trauma. In this case, the patient had felt so well for such a long time that she had ceased to be careful of how she was lifting things and using her back. She simply overdid it.

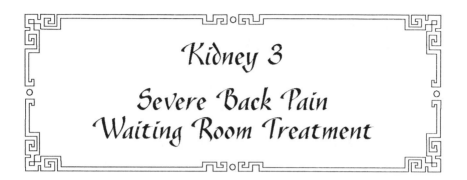

Kidney 3
Severe Back Pain
Waiting Room Treatment

Male, Age 38

On one very busy summer day, a thirty-eight-year-old man came in for an acute low back pain problem. He had injured his back while doing some yard work. All of the clinic treatment rooms were full, and there were other patients in the waiting room; but his pain was so severe that he was treated right there on the spot.

Upon examination, the pain was centered in the sacroiliac joint and was aggravated by the movement of his leg. For treatment, the Ling Ku combination was chosen. (Please see our first book, *Twelve and Twelve in Acupuncture*, for more information regarding this point combo.) Since the pain was mostly one sided (on the left), the right side was chosen to be needled. Unfortunately, the Qi sensation proved to be too strong for him in a sitting position, and he fainted. The needles were immediately removed and he was placed in a lying position on the floor. The points Du 26 and Stomach 36 were massaged, and he regained consciousness in about 1 minute. He reported a slight improvement in the pain, but it was still intense. He was made more comfortable on the floor, with pillows beneath his head and knees. A needle was inserted on the right side at Kidney 3, with a gentle but continuous stimulus administered for 2 to 3 minutes. The pain decreased enough so that he was able to stand up without assistance, something he had not been able to do a few minutes earlier. He returned for treatment the next day, with some improvement. He was treated in a lying position, with the Ling Ku combination and KD3 on the right, Lung 7 and Urinary Bladder 60 on the left. This treatment was repeated three times a week for a total of seven treatments. He has experienced no recurrence to date.

Summary

Kidney 3, with or without the Ling Ku combination, can be dramatically effective in treatment of acute sacroiliac pain. As illustrated by this case, distal points such as Ling Ku can generate a powerful Qi sensation, so care should be taken with patients if they become light-headed or faint. Even if only a few needles are used, the resulting Qi sensation might still be too strong for the patient.

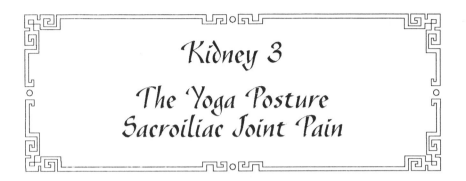

Kidney 3

The Yoga Posture
Sacroiliac Joint Pain

A thirty-five-year-old male yoga enthusiast, who had been receiving acupuncture treatment for a variety of health concerns, came in for treatment of a painful area around the sacroiliac joint. When performing certain yoga postures, the pain would be aggravated and radiate up into his lumbar region, especially on the left side around the fourth and fifth vertebrae. He first noticed the condition several weeks previously, and it had deteriorated since then.

Initially, he was treated with the Ling Ku combination (see references for this point combination in *Twelve and Twelve in Acupuncture*, pp. 14, 15, 38–47). In typical fashion, the points were needled on one side only and the left side was indicated. This treatment cleared the lumbar pain, but some of the sacroiliac joint pain was still present, reduced from a sharp pain to a dull ache. At this time, another point was added—Kidney 3. It was needled on the affected right side, and a strong sensation was obtained that radiated down into the bottom of his foot. The point was given a strong and continuous stimulus for about 1 minute, at which time the pain totally subsided. The needles were left in place for about 30 more minutes, being stimulated three more times at about 10 minute intervals. He received two more treatments the following week after which the pain ceased to recur, unless an extra strenuous yoga practice aggravated it again.

Summary

This case provides us with another example of a condition that is reaggravated by a specific activity, and the need to avoid such activity until the problem is completely cleared up. The patient was convinced that yoga was good for him—however, certain positions caused an excessive amount of force to be placed on his lower back, and the result would cause pain in his sacroiliac joint. In this case, convincing him of the need for moderation, even in his yoga practice, was the key to his eventual recovery.

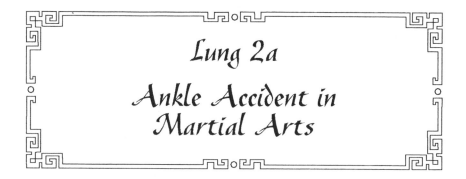

A martial artist tripped during his class, badly spraining his ankle. He was 38 years old and otherwise in good health. After seeing little improvement following a week's rest, he decided to come in for acupuncture treatment.

Upon observation, the right ankle was swollen and tender to the touch, particularly along the line between Urinary Bladder 59 to 61. Dorsiflexion and extension were severely limited. The achilles tendon felt hard and rigid upon palpation. A very sensitive ah shi spot was located in the area surrounding Lung 2 on the left side.

For treatment, only this LU2 ah shi was used; it was needled on the left side only, with a 30 gauge needle. A strong Qi sensation was obtained, and in conjunction with stimulation of the needle he was told to try moving his ankle.

To his amazement, he found it possible to move his ankle much more than before. He was left to rest with the needle in place, and periods of stimulus were given every 10 to 15 minutes. The total time of the first treatment was 45 to 50 minutes. At the conclusion of this treatment, some liniment was applied along with some light Tui Na, to help with the blood and Qi stagnation. He was encouraged to use some herbal plasters he had at home. Upon returning the next day, he reported still feeling the effect of his latest acupuncture treatment. In all, he estimated the degree of improvement as being in the neighborhood of 60 to 70 percent. He was treated daily in this fashion with continuing progress for 5 more days. At the end of the five days, he guessed his improvement to be around 80 to 90 percent. He was treated three more times the following week until he reported experiencing no further pain, at which time his treatment was discontinued. He went back to his martial arts class and resumed working out. He has experienced no recurrence to date.

Summary

Dr. Tan has found that the LU2 and the surrounding zone corresponds to the Tai Yang area of the ankle. Treatment is administered at the ah shi site. In most cases, the LU2 ah shi is found slightly lateral to the classic point location, into the medial portion of the deltoid muscle.

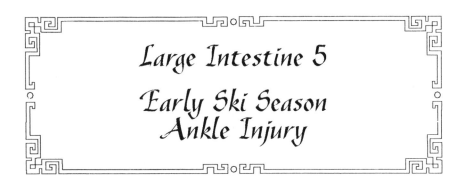

Large Intestine 5

Early Ski Season Ankle Injury

Male, Age 28

An avid sports enthusiast and skier, this patient injured his left ankle . . . unfortunate just at the beginning of ski season. It was severe enough to warrant x-rays at the ski resort's emergency room. The x-rays were negative for bone fracture, so his injury was diagnosed as severe sprain and strain of the ankle, with possible ligament damage. Back in San Diego, he decided to see if acupuncture could help speed his recovery. Aside from his ankle, he presented with no other obvious health problems, appearing fit and athletic in build.

Upon examination, the ankle was visibly swollen—the most noticeable area being in the zone around Stomach 41 and Gall Bladder 40. Attempting to dorsiflex the foot aggravated the pain, causing it to radiate upward along the lateral side of the tibia, occasionally all the way to the knee. He could also detect some stiffness in the lateral part of his knee at these times. Rotation of the ankle was somewhat limited in range, but did not aggravate the pain very much. Thus it was determined that the principle channel involved was the Yang Ming of the foot.

For treatment, Large Intestine 5 was selected to treat the ankle, with LI11 added to address the knee injury. (Please see *Twelve and Twelve in Acupuncture* for more information on LI11 and knee pain.) The two points were connected together with an electronic-stimulator, set at a low frequency (1–3 cps.) regular rhythm. The treatment lasted approximately 45 minutes, at the end of which he found that he could flex his ankle more without feeling any pain. He estimated his improvement as being halfway there, or about 50 percent; yet he was still unable to put all of his weight on it for an extended period of time.

Unfortunately, he was unable to come in every day for treatment, (an ideal protocol for acute injury), so he was treated three times a week. He came in for his second treatment 2 days later feeling much improved, having traded his crutches for a cane. The same treatment was administered, with further improvement noted. At the time of his third treatment, less than a week later, he was no longer bothered by stiffness or discomfort in his knee; the only point employed was LI5, needled deeply towards San Jiao 4. After this treatment, the pain had decreased further, and the range of motion had visibly increased. After the seventh treatment, he had regained full range of motion, but was still unable to put all of his weight on the ankle for any length of time. Impressed with his own pro-gress, he agreed to continue treatment in an effort to completely recover. After another seven treatments he was able to walk normally, without pain. He subsequently went back to skiing, with no further problem from either his ankle or knee. The total length of time from his injury to complete recovery from this severe ankle problem was about 5 weeks.

Summary

This case provides another example of what might be our distal treatment method's forte—its use in "Sports Acupuncture." A freshly sustained injury is often contraindicated for local needle treatment. A distal method is often the only kind that can be employed safely, and as in this case, effectively.

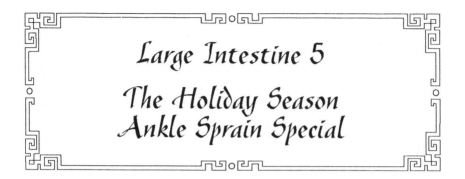

Large Intestine 5
The Holiday Season
Ankle Sprain Special

Female, Age 38

This patient called Dr. Tan at home on Christmas Day, because she had sprained her ankle. Unfortunately, he was out of town for a couple of days. In the meanwhile, she sought treatment from another acupuncturist, who administered a treatment consisting mainly of local points with heavy stimulation. The treatment had no effect, and the next day her ankle felt even worse. The following day Dr. Tan returned, and was able to see her within hours of getting back in town.

On observation, the right ankle was clearly swollen, with most of the distention evident along the Stomach and Gall Bladder channels. The range of motion was extremely limited, almost nil, and she was unable to stand on it with more than 50 percent of her weight.

For treatment, Large Intestine 5 was selected and needled on the left side. The needle was inserted deeply in the direction of the joint, almost to the point San Jiao 4.

124

As might be suspected, a strong Qi sensation was obtained, at which time she was told to try moving her ankle around. To her surprise, she was able to move her ankle in flexion and extension a bit, something she had been totally unable to do just minutes before. The period of stimulus was approximately 30 to 45 seconds, after which she was left for a while to let the Qi work. The needle was stimulated for a similar length of time at approximately 5 to 10 minute intervals. The treatment itself lasted about an hour, with the patient experiencing considerable relief from the pain.

There was, however, no discernible reduction in the degree of swelling around her ankle. In instances such as this, involving new acute injuries, treatment should be given more frequently. In this case daily treatment was called for. The next day, following her second treatment, she reported feeling more than 50 percent better, with a visible reduction in the ankle swelling. In all, she was treated for 5 consecutive days, LI5 being the only point employed to address her ankle injury. She was treated one more time at the beginning of the next week; at this time it became clear that she required no further treatment for this problem. She has experienced no further difficulty with her ankle since then.

Summary

This was a case in which the standard channel theory as taught in most acupuncture colleges failed to work. By modifying this theory and applying it contralaterally, a good result was obtained. Further effectiveness was derived by connecting the corresponding two channels involved—the foot Yang Ming and the foot Shao Yang—with a single needle from LI5 to SJ4. This approach often works as well as it did here all by itself, but on occasion it may be necessary to also treat locally. In such a case, we find it is usually best to open with stimulating the distal points while the patient moves the affected area, then to treat locally for a while, and to finish by removing all local needles and repeating the opening procedure again. Usually the second attempt to move the injured area will produce more mobility and less pain.

Chapter 5
Final Considerations

USE THIS INFORMATION

Now that you have read about the specific usage of the twenty-four points, please try them out! The effectiveness of this distal point method will never be fully realized if practitioners do not put it to the test in their clinics.

THE FEEDBACK FORM

We all learn from each other. We learn from our teachers, of course, but we also learn from our students when we teach—and we learn from our patients as we treat them. As authors, we want to have the opportunity to learn from our readers. We really appreciated the response that we received from the "Feedback Forms" that were returned to us from the first book, *Twelve and Twelve in Acupuncture.* We are again including a "Feedback Form" for you to fill out and return to us. Please also take the time to let us know how you pesonally feel about our work.

SEMINARS AND WORKSHOPS

Since the publication of our first book, we have become increasingly involved in giving seminars and workshops based upon our books and articles. We are committed to making the time to do so in the future. We plan to have several continuing education events every year in the San Diego area, as well as a number of 1 and 2 day seminars in various cities around the country.

FUTURE PLANS

Following the publication of *Twenty-Four More in Acupuncture*, will be other related works, many that deal entirely with practical clinical information. However, we do plan to publish a text focusing on the several theories that Dr. Tan has drawn upon to produce much of his clinical expertise. Feedback from our readers will play a big part in helping us formulate a plan for upcoming publications . . . so please let us know what topics are of interest to you.

Bibliography

Acupuncture: A Comprehensive Text. Shanghai College of Traditional Medicine. Seattle, Washington: Eastland Press, 1981.

Chinese Acupuncture and Moxibustion. Beijing, China: Foreign Language Press, 1987.

Twelve and Twelve in Acupuncture. Richard Tan and Stephen Rush: San Diego, California, 1991.

Index 1
Point Descriptions and Case Studies

———•◦•———

Point descriptions and applications are in bold type.
Case studies for each point are in regular type.

Index 2
Symptoms and Conditions

———•◦•———

Visit Dr. Tan's website at **www.DrTanBalance.com**:

- Register for classes online

- Plan for upcoming seminars

- Participate in the on-line forum

- Learn about Ba-Zi (Chinese Astrology)

- Discover Feng-Shui tips to enrich your environment

- Order Dr. Tan's books on Acupuncture & Feng Shui

    – *Twelve and Twelve in Acupuncture*
    – *Twenty-Four More in Acupuncture*
    – *Shower of Jewels*
    – *Dr. Tan's Strategy of Twelve Magical Points*
    – *Acupuncture 1, 2, 3*

To order books by mail, you may write to:

Office of Dr. Richard Tan
4550 Kearny Villa Road, Suite 107
San Diego, CA 92123

NOTES